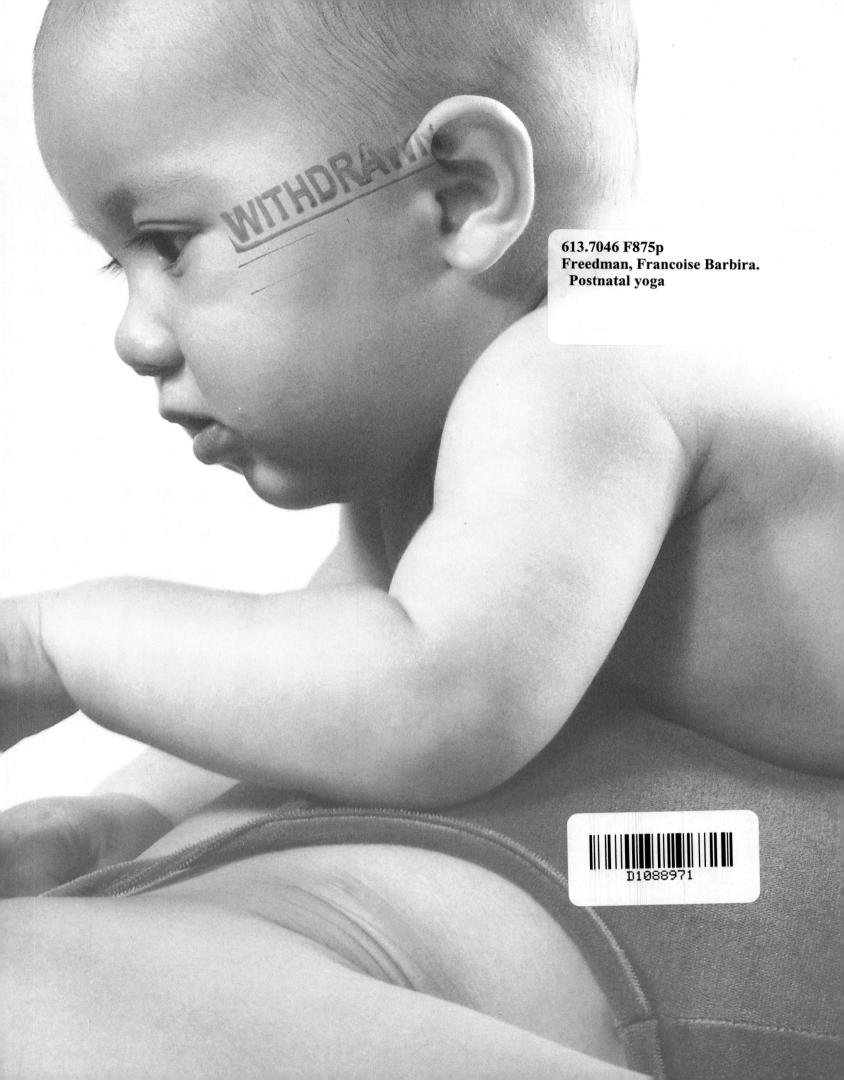

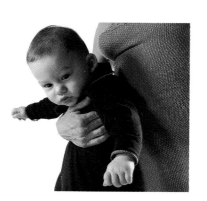

Postnatal Yoga

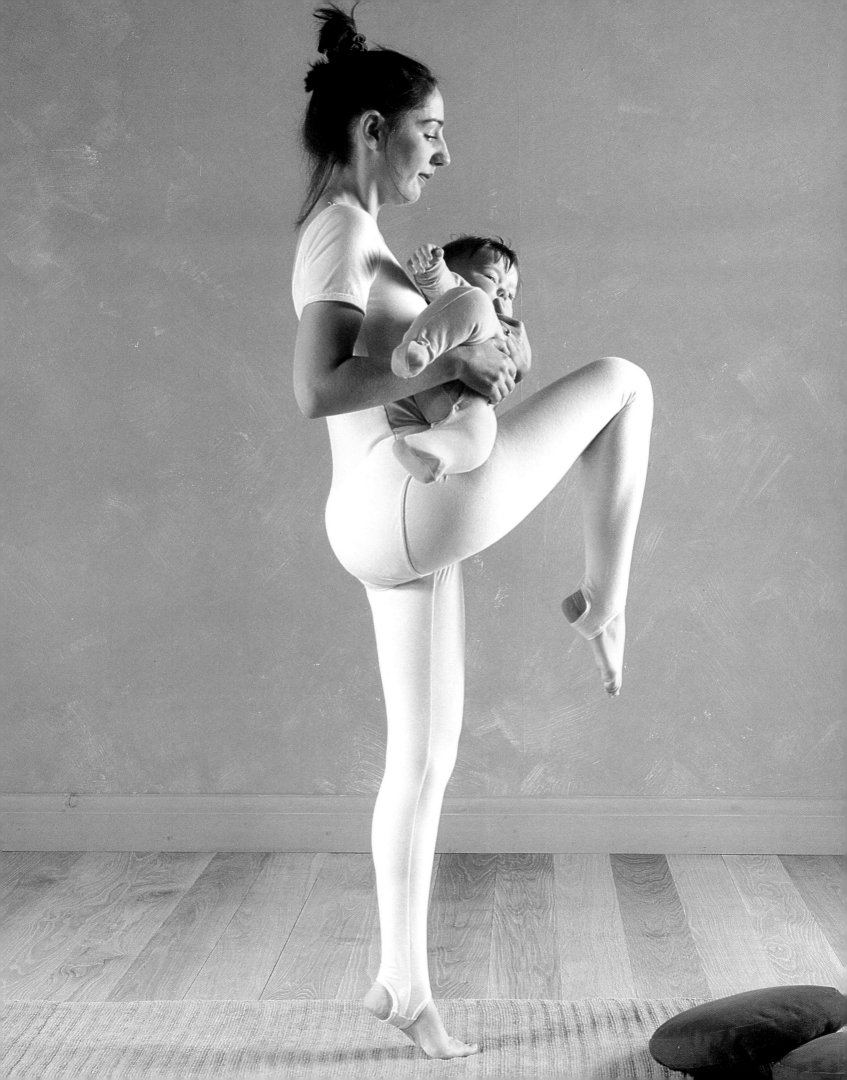

Strengthening
body and spirit
after birth –
a guide for new
mothers

Postnatal

Yoga

françoise barbira freedman
with doriel hall

photography by christine hanscomb

LORENZ BOOKS

For Mary, "little peach"

First published in 2000 by Lorenz Books

Lorenz Books is an imprint of
Anness Publishing Limited
Hermes House
88–89 Blackfriars Road
London SE1 8HA

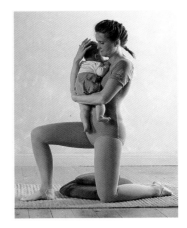

Published in the USA by Lorenz Books,
Anness Publishing Inc., 27 West 20th Street,
New York, NY 10011; (800) 354 9657

This edition distributed in Canada by
Raincoast Books
8680 Cambie Street
Vancouver
British Columbia V6P 6M9

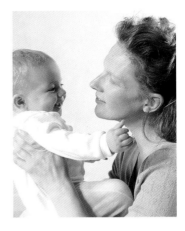

A CIP catalogue record for this book is available
from the British Library

Publisher: **Joanna Lorenz**
Project Editor: **Debra Mayhew**
Designer: **Lisa Tai**
Photographer: **Christine Hanscomb**
Production Controller: **Don Campaniello**

10 9 8 7 6 5 4 3 2 1

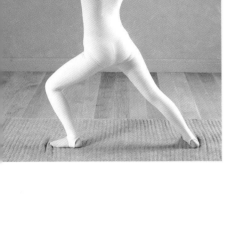

Publisher's note: The reader should not regard the
recommendations, ideas and techniques expressed and
described in this book as substitutes for the advice of a
qualified medical practitioner or other qualified
professional. Any use to which the recommendations,
ideas and techniques are put is at the readers sole
discretion and risk.

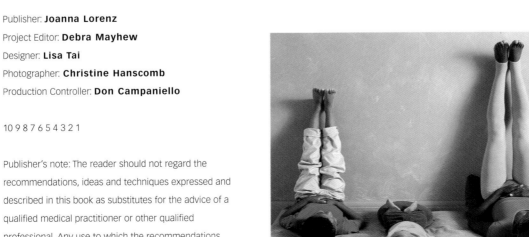

Contents

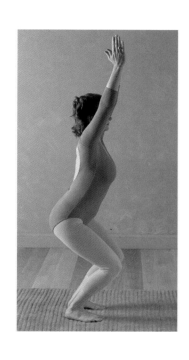

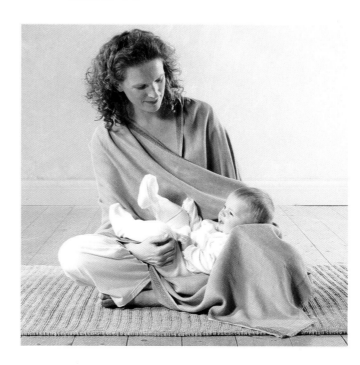

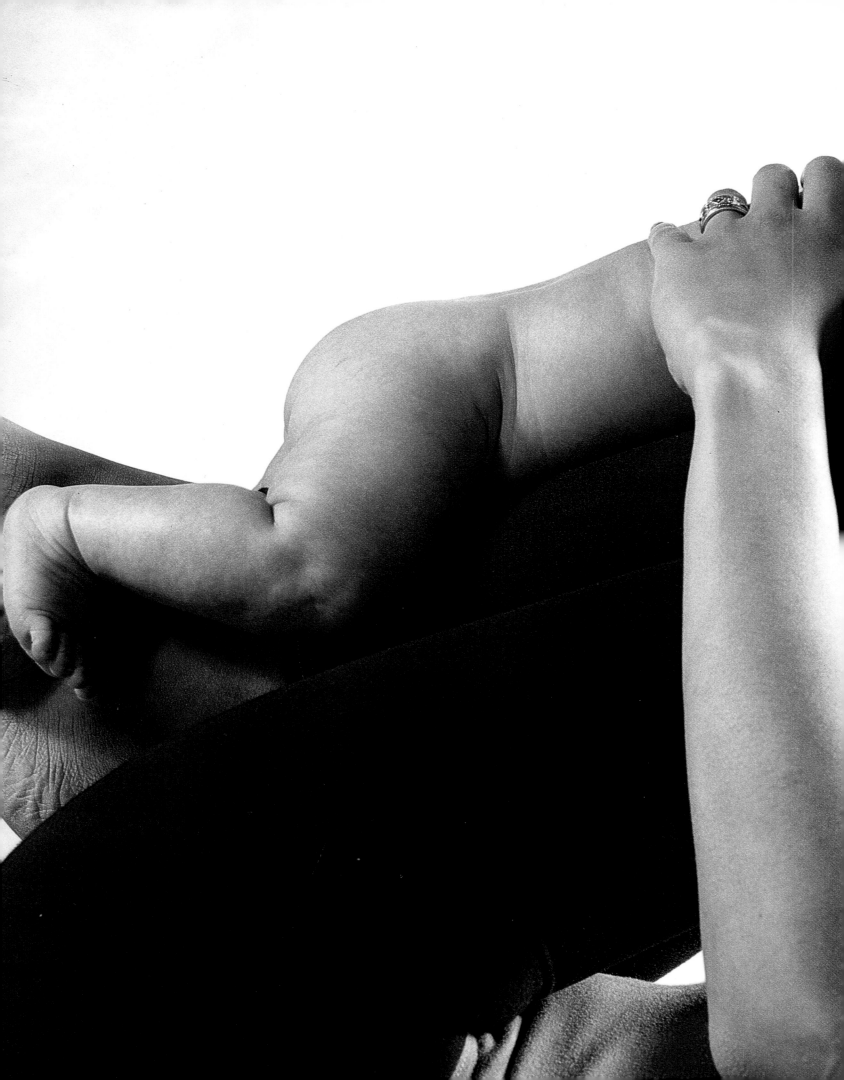

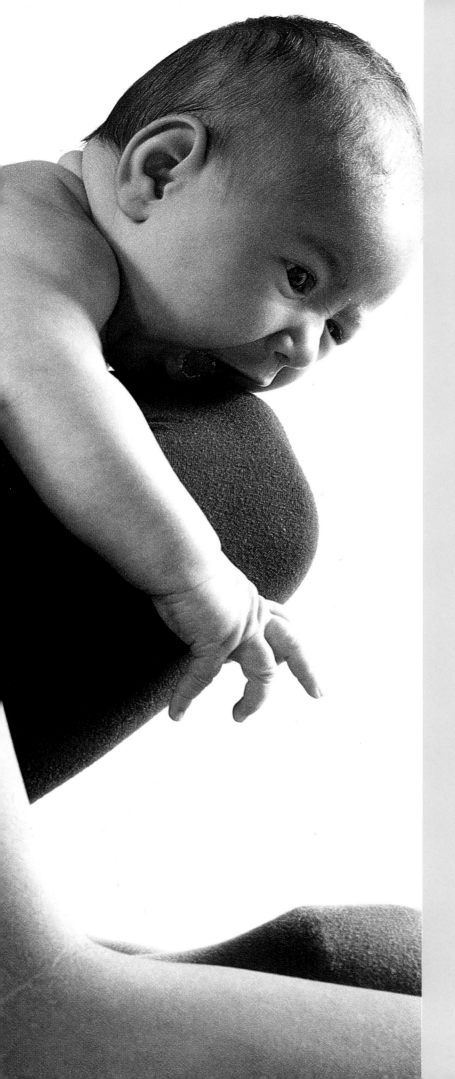

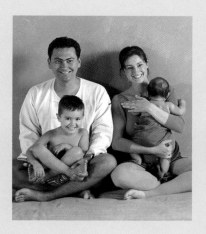

introducing
yoga

Giving birth transforms women's lives in
profound, and often unexpected, ways.
Each experience is different, and yet all
births call for a new integration of physical
and spiritual well-being. The flow of breath
in yoga opens a steady calm path in the
midst of all the emotions and changes that
new mothers inevitably go through.

birthing lightly with yoga

So here you are, at home with your new baby. Congratulations!

Giving birth can be a very demanding physical event. It can also give rise to strong emotional and spiritual experiences. Who can gaze at a tiny baby without being stirred by feelings of joy and awe at the miracle of new life? When the baby is your own newborn, such joy may be accompanied by feelings of apprehension. The well-being of this helpless child depends upon your ability to nurture him or her, to satisfy his or her needs.

Yoga can give you much-needed support at this time of changing responsibilities. Yoga is an ancient system of self-help that helps bring health and a feeling of "lightness" into every level of your being – physical, emotional, mental and spiritual. Regular yoga practice will quickly increase your overall feelings of health and fitness. You will grow stronger, more confident, calmer, and better able to nurture your baby, as well as the other members of your family. You will experience and be able to spread real happiness as you nurture yourself and those close to you.

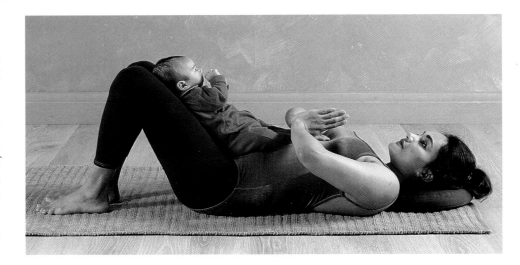

yoga with birthlight

You may have been practising yoga for years, or perhaps you discovered it during your pregnancy. If so, you will already know what an enormous help yoga can be in any demanding situation. Birthlight is a practice of yoga that enables women to "birth lightly", making use of the breath to increase the efficacy of uterine contractions in labour. It allows you to release fear and tension while your baby is born.

◁ **Keep your baby near you during yoga practice. He or she will enjoy watching you, and will be safe and comfortable lying close by you on the floor, propped up on cushions or a beanbag. This is also an ideal place for your baby to fall asleep while you are doing your yoga practice.**

△ **Lie on your back with your knees bent, feet flat on the floor. Pressing your hands together, breathe as deeply as possible. Each inhalation will tone and strengthen your back muscles.**

yoga is for everyone

If you are absolutely new to yoga then this is a wonderful time to start, just when you need all that it has to offer you to adjust to the joys and challenges of motherhood.

Whether this is your first, second or third baby – or if you have just had twins – the exercises and advice given in this book will help you. They have been specially designed to address your needs as a new mother, and take you safely from the earliest days after giving birth towards full personal fitness and confidence in your maternal role.

this book is for you

The following pages will lead you gradually through exercises which are designed for you to acquire increased pelvic strength and long-term pelvic health. The programme starts with the underlying core elements of yoga: awareness, breathing, relaxation, positive attitude and physical stretching. To this core are added, as the weeks and months after the birth flow by, progressively more vigorous and demanding postures and asanas (classical poses). Each exercise is numbered so that you can refer easily to the

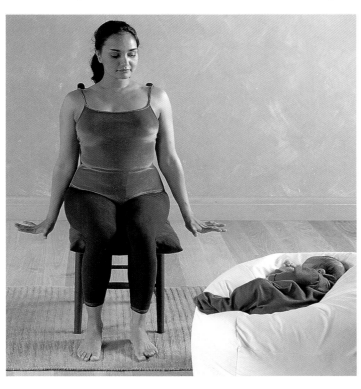

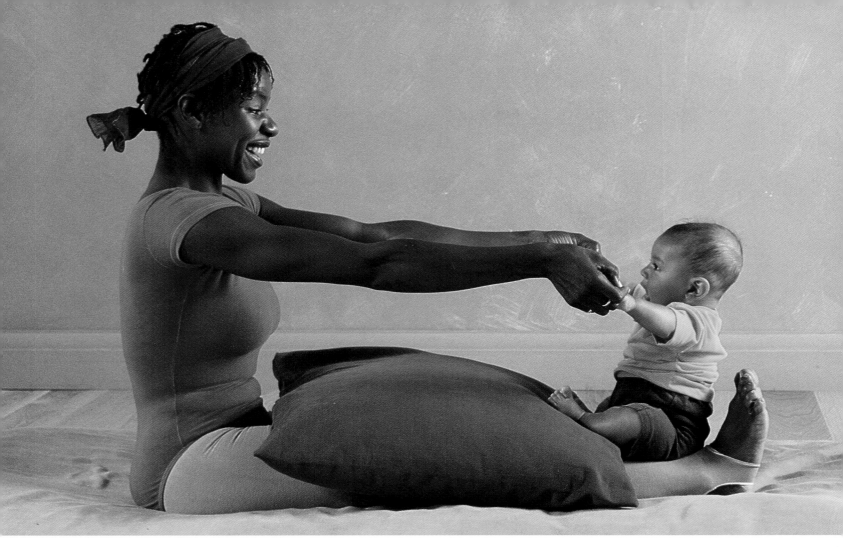

△ **Sit upright as often as possible, first against a wall and then without support to strengthen your lower back. Feel a straight line from your crown to your seat.**

earlier stages of each exercise as you develop and strengthen the posture over time. This progression will encourage you to keep the suppleness that comes with pregnancy and to add to it increasing strength and stamina.

Use the book to suit your own needs and those of your baby or babies. Each family is different, of course, but every resourceful and determined new mother can find a few moments, several times each day, to practise the movements, the breathing exercises and the relaxations that are shown in this book: you will find that it is time well spent.

Involve the family. Have fun together. Be lighthearted. Yoga brings "lightness" to mind and body, and spreads it all around.

▷ **Sitting cross-legged is a comfortable position to do your yoga breathing while playing with your baby. Try to keep your spine straight and you will feel the benefits of this stretch.**

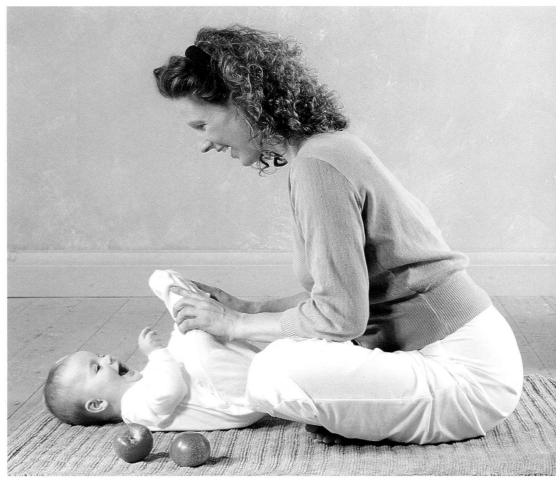

The essence of yoga

Yoga is a holistic system. It is based upon the belief that the physical, emotional, mental and spiritual levels of your being interact within the "energetic aspect" that is the invisible double of your physical body. This aspect has its own interconnecting pathways. The main channel passes, like a motorway, through the energetic aspect of the physical spine. It has "junctions" along it, like roundabouts, where "energy traffic" joins and leaves the channel. Many healing traditions refer to these junctions as the Chakras – this means "wheels", "vortices" or "roundabouts".

Therefore, anything that influences the flow of energy affects you at every level. Your physical body contains and processes three main types of energy – "life", "love" and "light" – which travel along the channel of the spine.

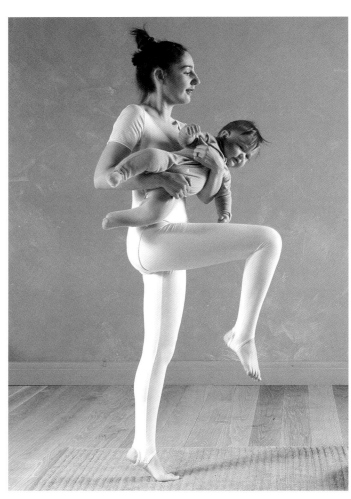

▷ **Lifting one bent leg allows you to extend your spine more, raising yourself on your toes before bringing the bent leg to the floor in a "tall walk".**

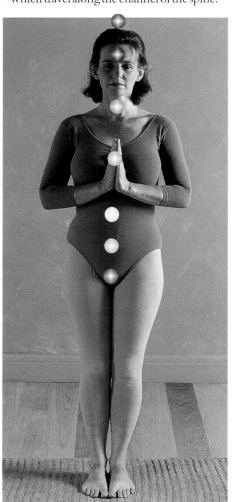

◁ **Standing in Tadasana (28), press your feet firmly on the floor and extend your spine to align your body again after giving birth. Be aware of your Chakras at all times.**

strength and vitality

Yoga enhances your physical vitality – this is the "life" aspect of energy – chiefly by involving the lower part of the body (the abdomen, lower back, legs and feet). Many of the strengthening yoga postures in this book are standing positions and lower back stretches. The gentle movements of yoga help to restore tone in the deepest muscles, to streamline the figure and to build up your strength and vitality after giving birth. Ensure that you exercise both sides of your body equally for overall balance. Begin on your right side then repeat the same number of movements on your left.

During pregnancy, your body was required to "open out" to accommodate your growing baby. Your abdominal muscles and pelvic floor muscles became very elastic, so that the baby could be born. All the emphasis in prenatal yoga practice was upon facilitating this opening and elasticity.

Now the situation is reversed. It is time to "close up" your body while maintaining and developing the physical suppleness and the openness of heart and mind that birth brought. This is a gradual process, but by about nine months after the birth you can expect to feel better than you felt before.

breath is the key

Yoga enhances emotional contentment – the "love" aspect of energy – chiefly by involving the middle part of the body (the upper back, chest, shoulders, throat, arms and hands). Yoga breathing exercises focus upon developing inner strength, stamina and your serenity, by acting upon the nervous system.

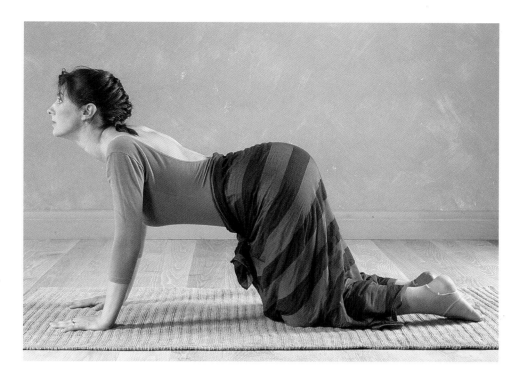

The breathing mechanism is linked to the nervous system, which controls how you feel. Because of this physiological link, the breath is the key to your sense of well-being. It is the only so-called "automatic" function of the body that you can learn to change at will.

As you gradually develop the habit of deep, slow breathing, you are encouraging your nervous system to make you feel good about yourself and your life. This is the yoga way to breathe. Fast, shallow breathing, on

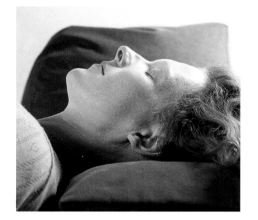

△ Relaxation gives you the deep rest essential to renew your energy.

the other hand, accompanies feelings of anxiety and stress. Indeed, if it becomes an ingrained habit it can actually engender these feelings, even when there is no obvious external reason for them. Negative feelings disappear when you learn to change the way you breathe. If they return, as they probably will at times, you can simply breathe them away again.

relaxation and centring

Yoga enhances mental focus and clarity, which form the "light" aspect of energy, chiefly by involving the upper part of the

body (the face, head and especially the brain). Physical balancing exercises and mental visualizations work to sharpen your senses and your mental focus, whereas deep relaxation gives your whole body-mind system a total rest and helps to compensate for the inevitable loss of sleep in the early days. Yoga teaches you to perceive life, and therefore to act, from a point of mental and emotional balance. When you are feeling anxious and under pressure you need first to regain this balance through yoga. You can be so much more effective when you are centred and relaxed in body, mind and heart. You will also be more in tune with the universal flow of life.

Yoga relaxation will help you to rest and unwind, so that you can enjoy your baby and your family life. Yoga helps you to feel happy, secure and lighthearted. Your own ability to relax teaches your baby how to relax as well, so that you can enjoy life together. In turn, this feeling influences and inspires the rest of your family. Physical, emotional, mental and spiritual well-being after giving birth requires that you learn to nurture yourself in deep relaxation. Only then can you truly nurture anyone else.

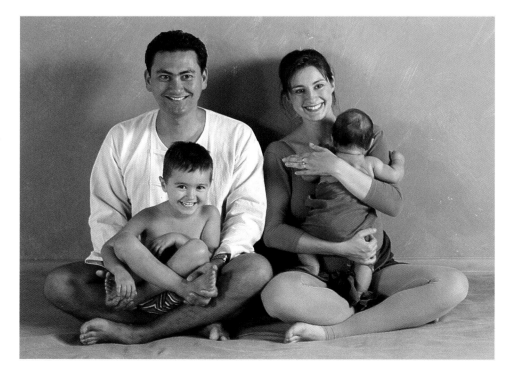

◁ Doing yoga together integrates the whole family and creates additional closeness. Yoga breathing can also help fathers to remain centred after the arrival of a new baby.

Yoga after giving birth

Your aim is to use the core aspects of yoga to bring you to a state of full health and vigour, starting from where you are now, soon after giving birth. You can expect to:
• Regain strength in the pelvic and abdominal regions.
• Relax and enjoy deep rest, to compensate for lack of sleep.
• Tone the body back into perfect alignment of hips and spine.
• Learn and practise self-nurture, so that you can nurture and enjoy your baby.

"Each birth, each baby,
each mother, is unique."

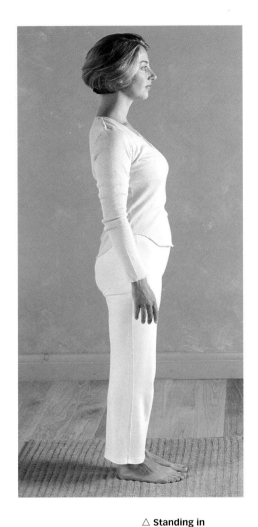

start at the beginning

Right now you may be feeling very well, or you may have all sorts of problems result-ing from hormonal imbalances, poor muscle tone or lack of sleep. However you are feeling, please start at the beginning of this book. The stages are carefully worked out to take you safely from your present postnatal state to your personal maximum level of well-being. Many of the problems that women face in later life – such as uter-ine prolapse or incontinence – can be traced back to lack of care after childbirth. They are usually avoidable, through an awareness of

posture and the right kind of progressive exercise after childbirth. Don't worry about your figure at this stage. It will be regained, perhaps improved, by inside toning.

posture

Regaining good posture is especially important after the birth. The abdominal muscles become very stretched during pregnancy. They may have been cut. Until they are healed and strengthened they cannot hold the spine firmly in place. New mothers need to take special care of the lower back.

△ **Standing in Tadasana (28), tilt your pelvis forward and backward slightly. Feel the link between your pelvic floor muscles and both your abdominal and lower back muscles.**

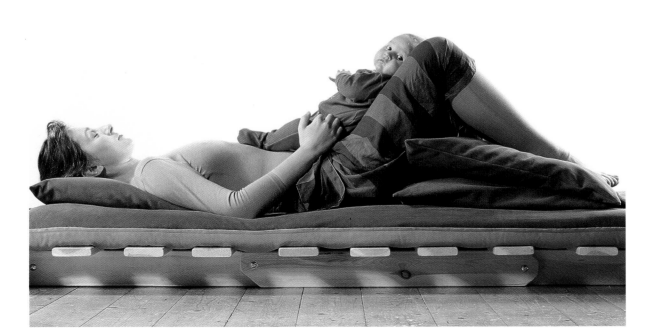

◁ **Use a futon or a firm bed, with cushions for extra support, for breathing and relaxation practice. It is comfortable for your baby, too.**

▷ As your baby grows and you regain strength, it is best to use an upright chair for breathing practice. Always make sure that your knees are level with your hips, using support to raise your feet if needed.

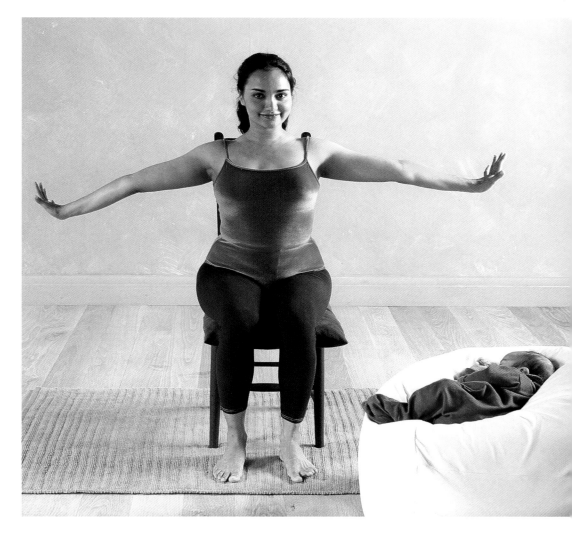

This book teaches you how to move with greater awareness, and to use your legs and upper back to sit and stand, to lift and carry. You then progress safely into gentle movements which build up into flowing sequences to gradually strengthen the weakened and overstretched muscles. Too much vigorous exercise, too soon, would simply strain them further. Full classical yoga postures should not be taken up until the after-effects of the pregnancy and birth have disappeared. It usually takes about six months to reach this stage.

what you need for yoga

Your body needs support, so that you are relaxed and comfortable as you practise. Keep a supply of cushions next to you. For breathing and relaxation you can use your bed, a futon, a firm armchair, or a long sofa. For movement and postures you will need a non-slip mat, measuring about 1 x 2m/3 x 6ft, that you keep just for your yoga practice. If you don't wish to buy one specially, you can use any suitable rug or piece of carpet.

Ideally, it is best to create a special "yoga space" in your home. This trains your mind in the yoga habit and helps you to maintain regular discipline. The good vibrations put you into the right frame of mind as soon as you enter this space, which makes it easy and enjoyable to settle down to regular practice and enjoy your progress.

You can practise relaxation after a heavy meal, but everything else is best done before a meal if possible, or after a light snack. Always wear loose clothes that do not constrict the abdomen, and take off your shoes and socks, so that energy can flow freely around your body.

You do not always have to find the time to install yourself in your "yoga space" or on a special mat or chair to practice yoga. If you cannot manage a practise that day, then just a few minutes of yoga can help you. No effort, no matter how small, is wasted in yoga. The aim of this book is to help you to integrate yoga into your daily life as a new mother, both in your home and outside it.

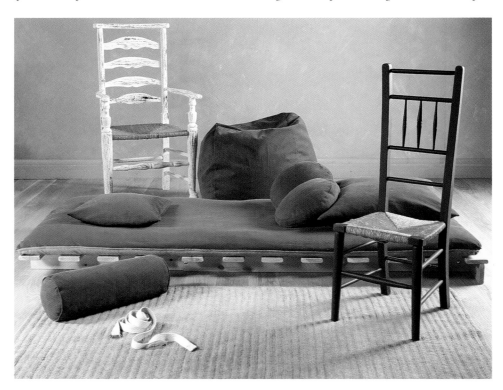

◁ A futon gives firm support for relaxation, and a beanbag and an upright chair will also be useful. Keep a special mat for your yoga practice. A belt can help your stretches.

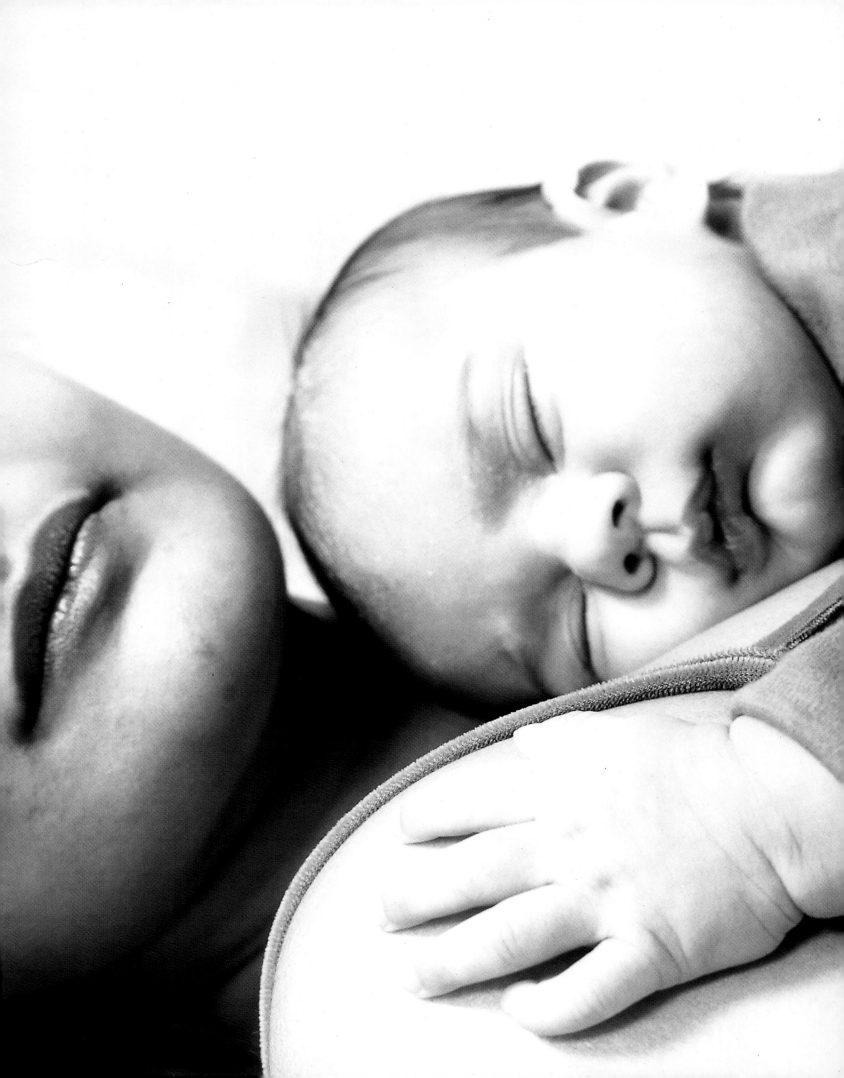

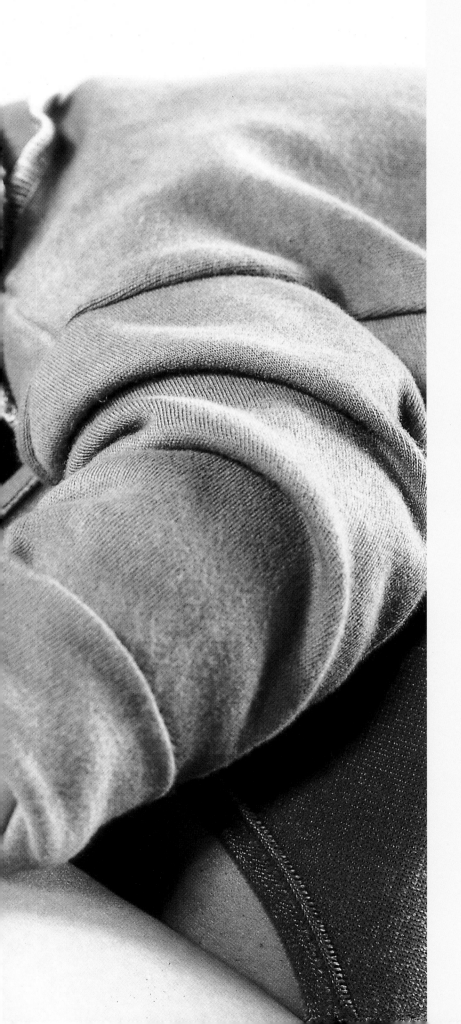

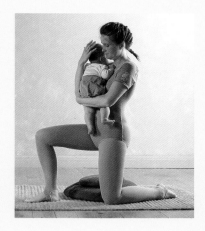

new
mothers

After the joy of welcoming your baby into the world, you may remember the firmer, slimmer body of early pregnancy and wonder if, when and how you will wear those clothes again. Trust the power of the breath in toning the deepest muscles in your body. They are your best allies to developing not only a fine figure but also your future strength.

Basic breathing techniques

Before you start any postnatal exercise, the first thing to focus on is your breathing. We call this "Yoga Breath Awareness". Watch yourself breathing. Become aware of your breath just as it is. Then, without forcing your inhalation, very gently extend your exhalation, allowing your natural breath to become gradually slower and deeper. This can have a profoundly calming and settling effect at any time. The breath is closely linked to the nervous system. Shallow breathing will make you physically tense, mentally distracted and emotionally anxious. Deep breathing has the opposite effect, making you centred and steady.

A deep breath in will quite naturally charge body and mind with new energy, and a deep breath out will release muscular tension, chemical waste products and feelings of tiredness and strain. For this reason, you should breathe deeply and slowly at all times during yoga practice, and the book will also give you guidance on when to breathe in or out. This joining of mind and body through breath and movement is yoga. After a few days' practice, you will be able to use your breath in many new ways.

You can use Alternate Nostril Breathing to energize and/or calm yourself, and Reverse Breathing to tone the deep muscle layers of your abdomen and spine. Take every opportunity to practise and perfect these breathing techniques. A good time to do this is while you are feeding your baby, as long as you can remain relaxed while you are practising.

1 Reverse breathing

During pregnancy you may have used breathing exercises to open the body, make more room for the growing baby and facilitate the birthing process. Now the situation is reversed: your aim is to close the lower part of your body, pull the stretched muscles inwards and upwards, and strengthen them so that they hold the spine, pelvis and abdominal organs in correct alignment. This is the purpose of Reverse Breathing. Practise for a few rounds, or until you feel tired or lose your rhythm. Stop and rest, and repeat whenever you feel ready. With practice, you will feel very toned and strengthened after breathing in this way.

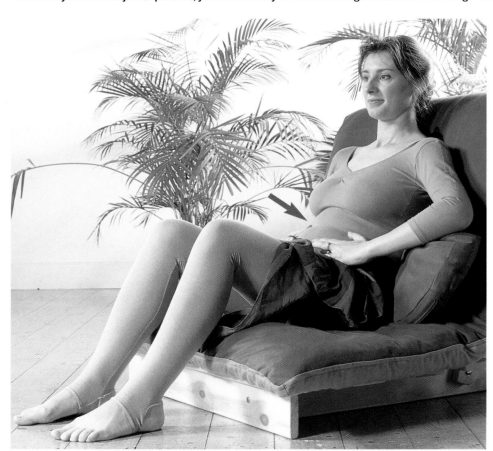

△ **1** Sit or lie comfortably, with your spine supported. Place your hands on your lower abdomen, to become aware of what is happening. Breathe in deeply, imagining the energy of the breath being drawn up through the base of your body into the abdomen.

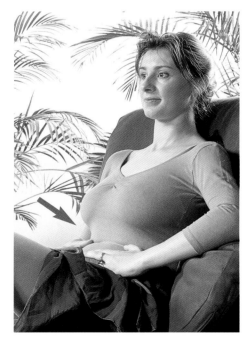

△ **2** As you breathe out, pull in your waist, drawing your navel up and closer to your spine at the back. Feel this out-breath continue to flow up into your chest, toning you powerfully from inside. Release at the end of your exhalation. The out-breath is longer than the in-breath, but this should never be forced. You can either take a "resting breath" in and out before inhaling and drawing up again, or repeat the Reverse Breathing without a pause.

2 Alternate nostril breathing

This exercise works on the nervous system, quickly soothing the emotions and calming the mind. Use it whenever you feel stressed, as well as part of your daily routine. Two complete breaths form one round: do several rounds. Your breathing will deepen naturally – never force it.

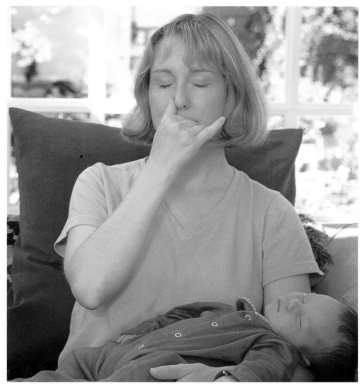

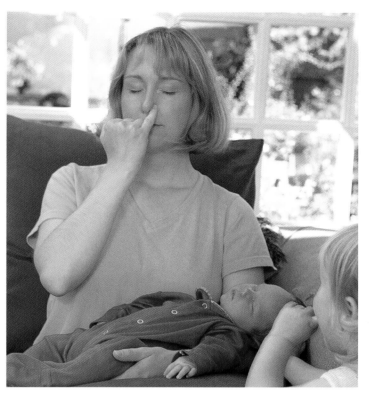

△ **1** Sit comfortably and erect. Bring your right hand in front of your face, with the three middle fingers tucked in towards your palm and the thumb and little finger extended. Place your thumb on your right nostril to close it, and breathe in through your left nostril.

△**2** Close the left nostril with your little finger and breathe out through the right nostril. Holding the hand position, breathe in through the right nostril, then close it with your thumb, open the left nostril by lifting your little finger and breathe out through it.

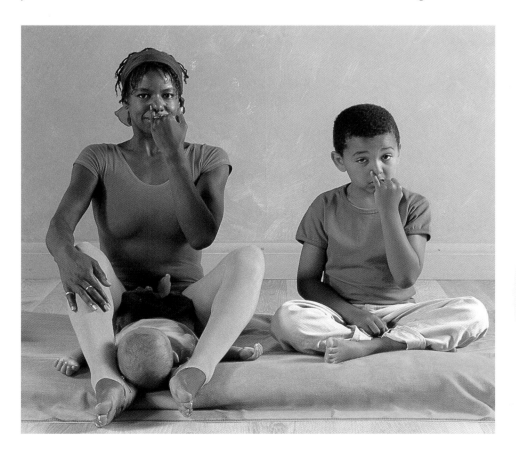

◁ **Whenever you feel the need for energizing, perhaps just after your baby has gone to sleep, a few rounds of Alternate Nostril Breathing will refresh you in two to three minutes. You can invite other children to do it with you before you play with them too.**

"The moment I first touched my new born, a love I had never felt before swept my heart."

Feeding and energy

You will enjoy your new baby most if you are feeling good in yourself. This good feeling largely depends upon two things: regaining your fitness and vitality, and being able to rest and relax despite the inevitable lack of sleep. Fitness and relaxation are the two keys to happy mothering and a happy baby, so these are the two "arms" of yoga that we will be focusing on in this book. Everyone in your family will enjoy the benefits of your yoga practice.

No sooner have you welcomed your baby into the world than feeding becomes an all-absorbing task. However well prepared you have been for this, it takes a great deal of adjustment for both your baby and yourself. Relaxing in a comfortable position can make a significant difference to your early experience of breastfeeding and make it more enjoyable from the start. If you are bottle-feeding, practising "yoga breath awareness" can contribute towards creating a closer physical bond with your baby.

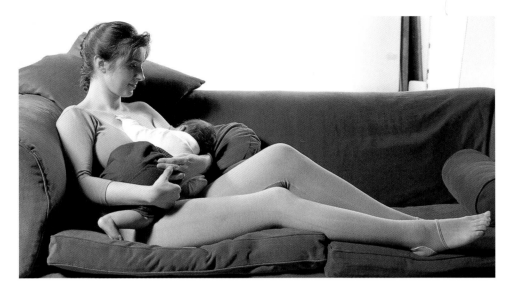

feeding positions

In the first weeks following birth, it is important that your back should always be well supported when you breastfeed. You may prefer a reclining position at first, in bed or on a sofa, but favour an upright position as soon as this is comfortable. If you have

△ While sitting up or reclined, make sure your lower back is well supported. Use a cushion to raise the baby's body if needed.

had a Caesarian section or a traumatic birth experience, lying down with your baby at your side may continue to be your most

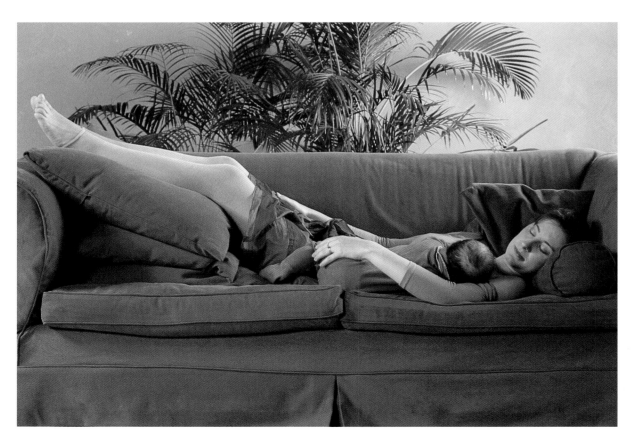

◁ If you had a Caesarean section you will need, at first, to find positions where the weight of your baby does not rest on your abdomen.

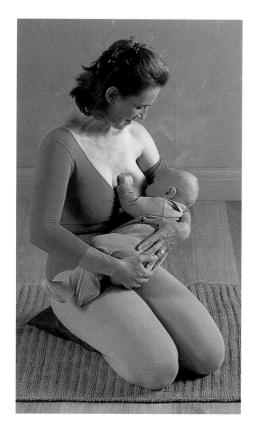

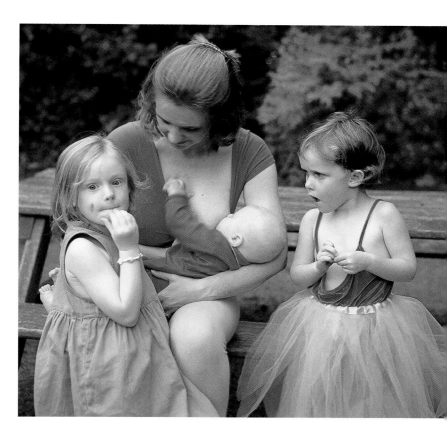

◁ As you grow stronger you will be able to feed your baby in a variety of positions. The important aspect is relaxed comfort.

▷ If you were in the middle of doing something else when the baby wakes for a feed, take a few deep breaths before you pick up your baby. This allows you to transmit a message of loving nurture to your baby, rather than one of irritation at being interrupted.

comfortable feeding position for longer. If needed, raise your baby on a cushion so that your back can remain straight while you feed. If you are sitting on a chair, you may need to place a cushion or use a support to raise your feet so that your knees and hips are level. Check your feeding position again and again, week by week, anywhere you happen to be with your baby, to make sure your back has adequate support while you feed. You spend so much time in feeding that forming good habits with regard to feeding positions is a fundamental step in regaining, or creating, a sound posture after birth. Always relax your shoulders.

breathing and relaxing while feeding

Feeding your baby is a precious time to practise breath awareness and save, if not generate, energy. Once you are settled in a comfortable position, use a deep exhalation to release any tension you hold in your body at the time. If you are breastfeeding, you can do this while the baby is "latching on" and

while hormonal changes are occurring in your body. Slow down your breath, using the "yoga breath awareness" technique, and feel that you are beginning to rest. If your baby does not feed easily and gets frustrated, start again calmly. Early obstacles can be overcome more easily and rapidly if you can break for relaxation while feeding your baby. Then feeding becomes a positive rest time in which you can practise some other breathing techniques, such as "reverse breathing", and also relax deeply while

remaining close with your baby. Making the best use of feeding times to renew and save your energy as a new mother is one of the main aspects of regaining fitness and vitality the yoga way.

bottle-feeding

It is even more important when bottle-feeding to breathe yourself into a welcoming, nurturing attitude before you pick up your baby. Relax while the baby is awake and alert at the beginning of the feed.

▷ Hold the bottle at a comfortable angle for your baby to suck on it. Relax and enjoy this moment of physical closeness and rest with your baby.

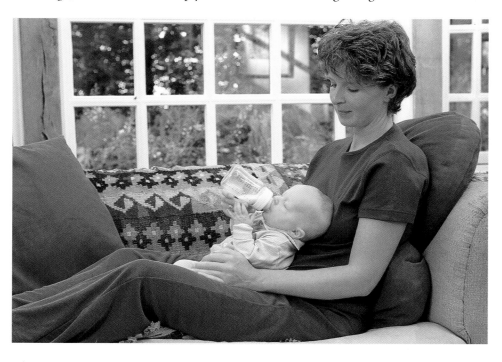

The art of relaxation

Yoga relaxation involves four elements: slow, calm breathing, comfortable posture, physical and mental relaxation. Slowing your breathing right down and breathing out slowly will calm the nervous system. You may already know, or will soon discover, how rapidly and well this works through your practice of expanded breathing. Relaxation is both a tool and a completion.

basic relaxation

In relaxation you do more than rest. You enter another state of being in which you are neither sleeping, nor engaged in activity. Think of it as putting your gearbox in the neutral position, disengaging from all your voluntary thinking and acting.

The more you stretch all the muscles of your body with yoga, the easier it becomes to relax them. The more you breathe in your stretches, the deeper your breathing becomes and the more you can make use of your breathing to either energize or quieten yourself. Life with a baby changes from day to day, nearly from moment to moment. Before you learn the classic yoga relaxation in Shavasana (27), or Corpse Pose, it helps to practise this basic relaxation whenever you can, through the day and night.

Although you will relax more deeply if you can lie down, any position in which you can settle comfortably for a minute or two is

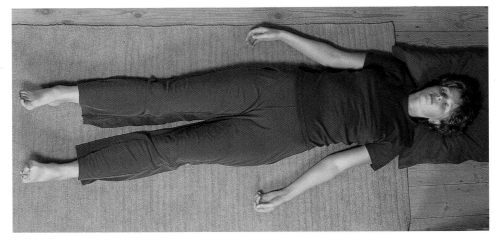

△ Lie on your back with your head, neck and spine in a straight line. Avoid letting your chin poke upwards by lengthening the back of your neck. Let your arms lie stretched out loosely, a little away from your body, with the palms up and fingers gently curled. The shoulders and upper back are spread wide and soft. Stretch out your legs, with your feet apart and rolling slightly outwards.

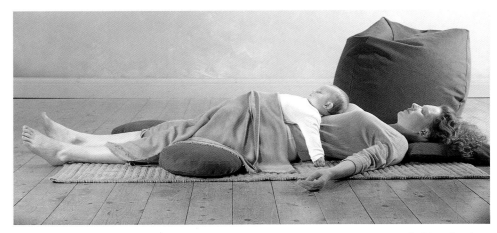

△ If you intend to relax deeply for ten minutes or more you may wish to cover yourself with a shawl (and socks in winter), as your body temperature will drop. Include your baby and relax deeply together.

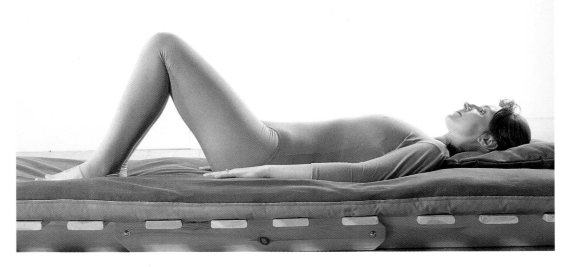

◁ If your pelvis tilts in this position, making a hollow under your waist, you may be more comfortable bending your knees and placing the soles of your feet flat on the floor to begin with, until in time your back remains flat with your legs outstretched. Meanwhile, press your back gently towards the floor as you breathe out.

▷ Once you have learnt how to make your body "let go" on demand, you can practise relaxation in many positions and situations. This is the Child Pose (67) which we look at later in the book.

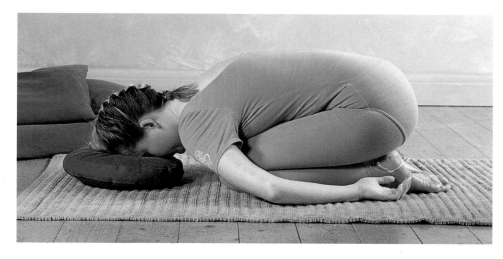

fine. Inhale, then extend the exhalation as much as you can. If you feel that you need to, then voice it, or Haaah, or yawn it, a few times. Then close your eyes and be aware of your breathing. If you have learnt to breathe in your abdomen while pregnant, feel yourself breathing deeply. Then let go of your conscious breathing and feel yourself resting. Experience the quality of rest that results from relaxing in stillness and quietening your breathing. At this stage you are entering the open space of relaxation, where your whole physiology can be refreshed and restored.

mental relaxation:
use the power of visualization

This aspect of yoga practice helps you to let go even more, releasing tensions within your body and also within your mind. Imagine yourself in a happy scene, such as lying in a beautiful garden. Build up this scene and make it very real for you. Bring your baby into your visualization. Feel close and bonded, with both of you basking in the sunshine of universal love, both

▷ Once you have learned the art of non-doing you can slip into this mode of being anywhere, any time you wish.

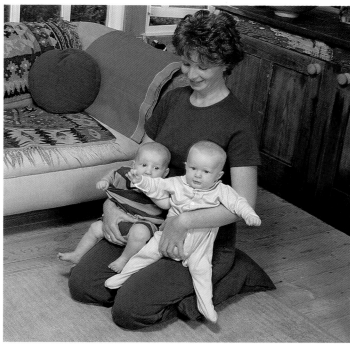

▽ Learning to relax and let go creates space for quality time with those we love.

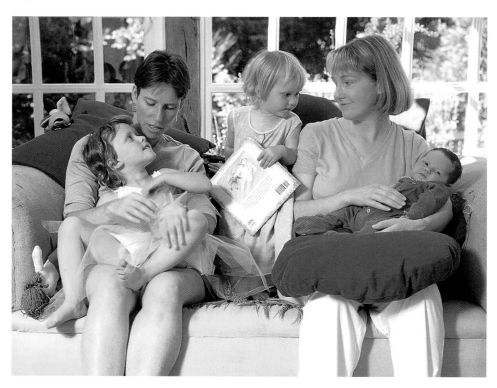

of you being nurtured together. Include others who are close to you in this happy scene. Feel loving and loved… After a while, let the vision fade away, knowing that it is always there for you to recapture. Focus on your breathing and start to come out of your relaxation.

emotional relaxation:
the attitude of surrender

This is the true purpose of your relaxation: to let go, to surrender to the flow of life, to be rather than to do. Learning to "go with the flow" makes a mother's life happier and her relationships more rewarding.

You can relax deeply while you are feeding your baby – to the great benefit of both of you. Use relaxation to help you to go back to sleep during disturbed nights, or to soothe your baby to sleep.

Breath, relaxation – and now movement

By increasing your awareness of your every-day movements, you can eliminate a great deal of postnatal tiredness and strain. Consciously allow your legs and upper back to carry your weight – and often that of your baby as well – rather than relying on your lower back and abdominal muscles. If you had a Caesarean section or episiotomy you will need to be especially vigilant while the scar tissue is healing. Practise the following exercises regularly, to restore muscle tone in the perineal and abdominal muscles. When these muscles are weak, the spine and pelvis move out of alignment, causing both poor posture and lower backache.

3 Reverse breathing II: for the pelvic floor

Practise the first stage of Reverse Breathing for a while, until you feel absolutely comfortable with it. Then add the following: as you breathe in, tighten and pull up the perineal muscles at the base of your body, drawing them up into the abdomen. Tighten the muscles at the centre of your "seat" (the vaginal muscles), drawing also on the back (anal muscles) and the front area (the muscles that hold your bladder in). This exercise, when practised regularly, can save years of discomfort and problems – including stress incontinence and prolapse – caused by perineal muscles that have been overstretched during childbirth.

Continue to tighten these muscles even more as you breathe, releasing them at the end of your out-breath. Practise using these sets of muscles in a smooth, wavelike flow of the breath. This exercise can be done almost anywhere and at any time. Rest for a few seconds between breaths, or between sets of six breaths. To alleviate any problems due to the weakness of your perineal muscles, do two sets of six breaths three times a day for two or three weeks.

4 Getting down to the floor and up off the floor

Getting down to the floor and up off the floor is something new mothers soon find themselves doing many times a day. If you have done yoga during pregnancy, you will already be familiar with the "all fours" position, called the "Cat Pose" (25). If not, why not start enjoying the benefits of this pose right away to soothe your back and avoid straining it as you go down to floor level and up again. This first basic sequence introduces yoga movement in your life as a new mother in a simple but effective manner. In yoga, body symmetry, suppleness and stretching are constantly practised so as to eventually become effortless during everyday activities.

▷**1** Once on the floor, position yourself on your hands and knees in a firm, symmetrical and well-balanced position "on all fours".

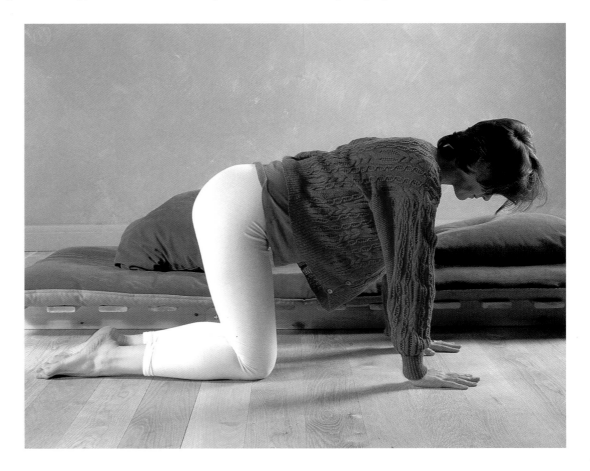

▷ **2** To get up off the floor, lean forward first so that you can easily turn your toes under. Then, in one flowing movement, walk your hands on the floor towards you while rolling your back to find yourself sitting on your heels, as shown. Remember to keep your neck relaxed.

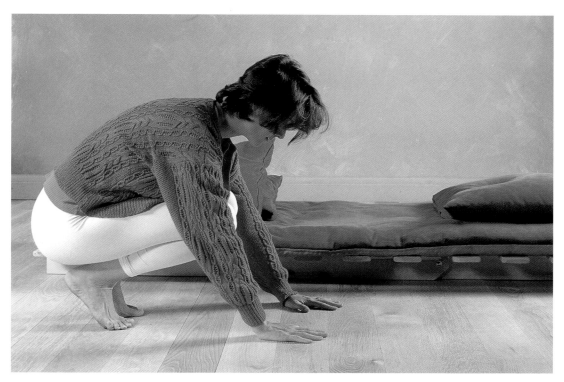

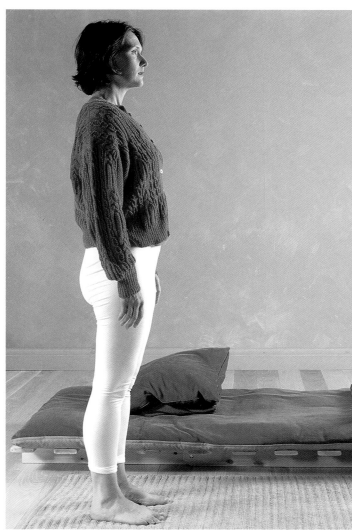

△ **3** By stretching your legs and pushing on your hands you find yourself getting up off the floor in one easy movement. With your legs bent at first, then extended, you can now stretch your spine to a full upright posture. Your lower back has been protected at all times during this sequence.

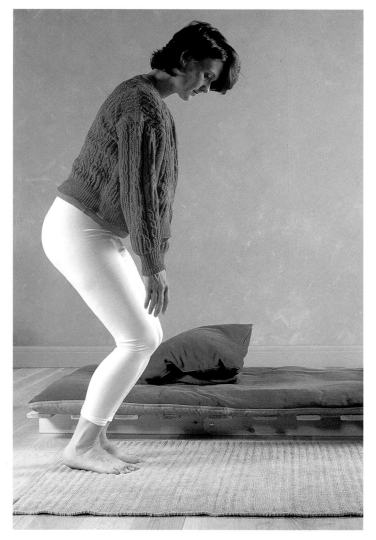

△ **4** Practise going down to the floor again on all fours by bending your knees and extending your arms towards the floor, palms stretched out. Your heels will probably lift from the floor as your knees reach down. Stretch on all fours and get up off the floor again, making this a rolling motion up and down.

Your first yoga routine

Every woman progresses at her individual rate, depending upon many factors: how well she is after the birth, how dedicated she is to her yoga practice, how busy her life is, and how well the baby is settling down. Some days flow smoothly whilst others seem to snarl up. The most important thing is to do what you can – today. Yoga is totally non-judgmental, so to compare yesterday with today is pointless. Every day is an opportunity to progress towards greater pelvic strength, better alignment of the spine, deeper relaxation, more serenity and inner balance. The weeks after giving birth bring huge changes, physically, emotionally and mentally. Your aim is to relax and heal, to energize and tone your body, your emotions and your mind. Regular deep breathing will keep you on course even when your emotions are all over the place. Above all, make time for rest.

If you have just a few minutes to spare, remember that relaxation comes before stretching. Alternate Nostril Breathing (2) is instantly relaxing – you will stretch all the better afterwards. If you are interrupted, take a few deep slow breaths to give your practice a completion.

yoga in the first six weeks

The routines here include postures on the floor (lying down, sitting and kneeling) and a few standing postures. Exercises can be practised on their own, or one page or more at a time.

Make sure that you do not do too much, too soon. The exercises included in this section are designed for the first six weeks after giving birth. You can continue, with great benefit, to do them for the rest of your life. But please do not go beyond them, to the next stage, until six weeks have passed. Even then, please wait if you do not feel ready for new challenges. It is far better to practise simple routines regularly, and to grow stronger and more relaxed, than to push yourself too fast and become stressed.

5 Legs up the wall

Even if the birth was relatively easy and you feel fit and well, take time to practise your Reverse Breathing (1) with your legs raised. If your birth was difficult, or you had a Caesarian section, it is important to tone your inner muscles with deep breathing. In the position below, the floor and wall will give you a solid support to help you to expand your abdominal breathing.

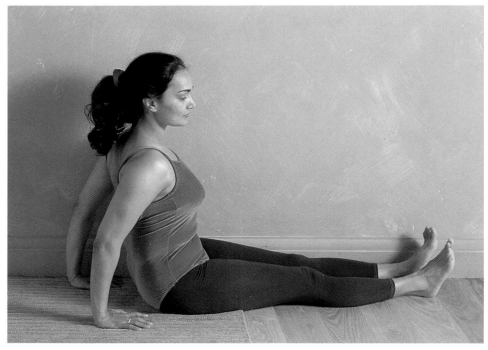

△ **1** Sit sideways against the wall. The aim is to place your legs parallel against the wall.

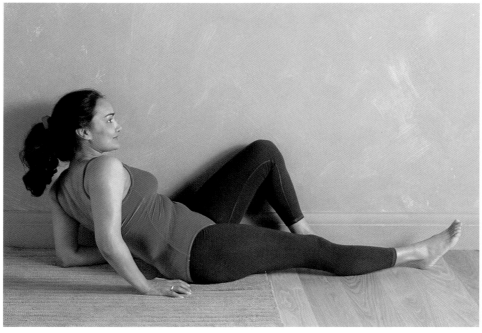

△ **2** Bend the knee nearest to the wall, leaning back on your hands.

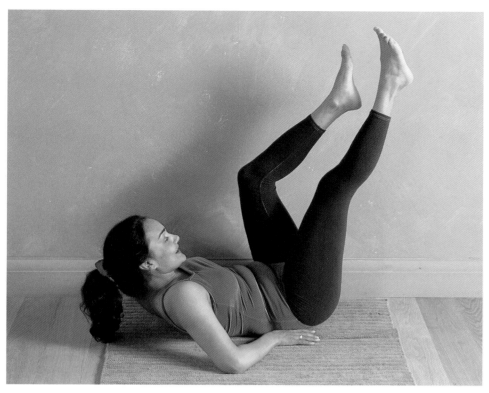

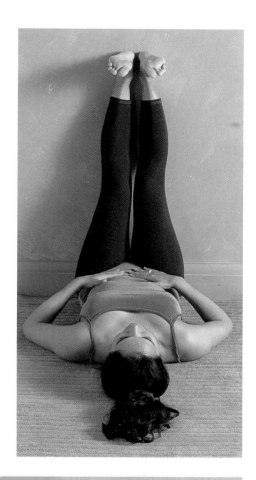

△ **3** Swivel round on your bottom, leaning back now on your forearms. Straighten your legs and move your upper body round.

▷ **4** You should be lying in a straight line with your legs together, hands on your abdomen. Flex your toes, lifting your heels, to strengthen your legs.

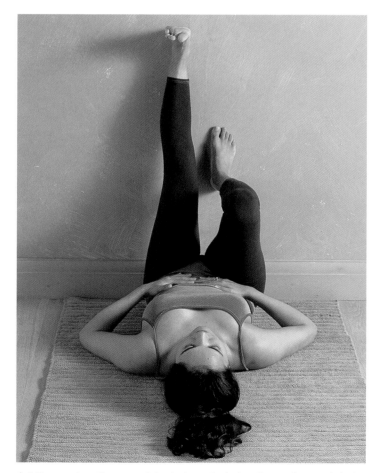

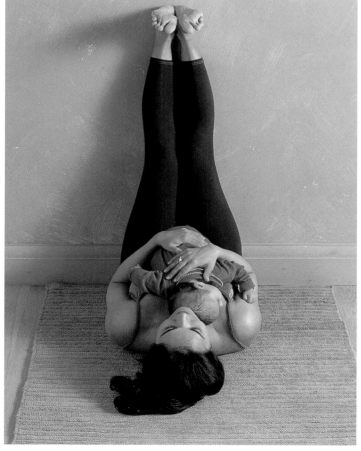

△ **5** You can strengthen your abdominal muscles by bending one knee and placing the sole of your foot on the wall, then repeating with the other leg. Remember that, after giving birth, you are working to close your body, so keep your legs together to tone your inner thigh muscles more effectively.

△ **6** Once settled in this position, you can include your baby. He or she will enjoy closeness with you, lying peacefully against your heart. Without even moving, you are using the calm power of your deep breathing to tone the lower back and abdominal muscles.

abdominal and lower back muscles

After your baby is born, lying flat on your back again is a new feeling. It is also the first, the safest and the best way to re-align your spine and tone the pelvic muscles in depth after giving birth. Feel your lower back settle into the floor and open up. One or both knees stay bent at all times to protect your lower back and ensure that you remain relaxed while you stretch. As your uterus returns to its normal size, yoga breathing allows toning through all the layers of abdominal muscles.

6 Knees to chest

In this exercise, Reverse Breathing (1) is used to tone the muscles of the lower back, together with the pelvic floor. Vaginal tone is also improved. If you have had a Caesarian section, do the first part – no. 1, below – only, for several weeks.

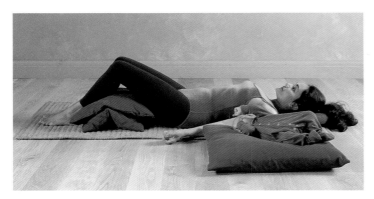

△ **1** Lie on your back with your knees bent and your feet flat on the floor. Stay comfortable and relaxed. Breathe freely in your abdomen.

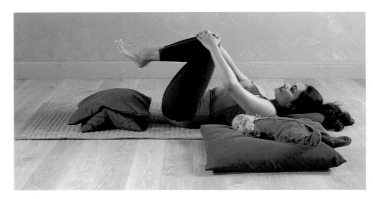

△ **2** Clasp your hands below your knees and, using Reverse Breathing (1), breathe in, drawing your pelvic floor muscles up, then further up as you exhale. Release.

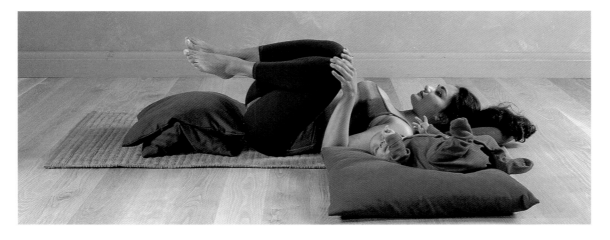

◁ **3** Inhale again and pull your thighs closer towards the chest as you breathe out, bringing your waist down towards the floor and widening your upper back. Repeat a few times.

7 Leg over

This exercise introduces a gentle twist which helps tone your transverse abdominal muscles as you practise your yoga breathing.

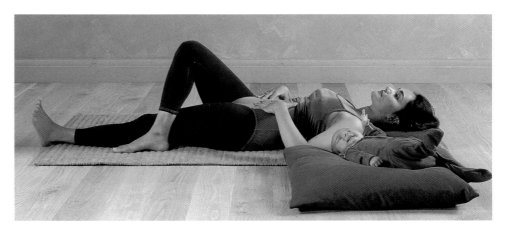

▷ Straighten one leg along the floor and place your other foot outside it, bending your knee. Place both hands on your abdomen. Breathe deeply, drawing your abdominal muscles in towards your spine as you exhale, and pressing your feet on the floor.

upper back and shoulder muscles

The exercises on this page aim to tone the dorsal muscles that were supporting your baby inside you, in your "bump". It may seem both enjoyable and strange to feel and regain ownership of this space with your yoga breathing. If your baby is awake you welcome him or her into your practice. Yes, baby, here you are, out in the world, but still close to your mother.

8 Hug yourself

This exercise helps to open your upper back and at the same time to recover the sense of your body as your own after giving birth.

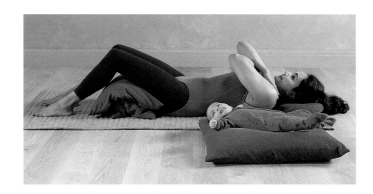

◁ Fold your arms across your chest, with fingertips on opposite shoulders. Hug yourself and breathe deeply, feeling the expansion in the back. As you exhale, press the base of your spine on the floor and let your whole back spread out.

9 Side stretch

This stretch elongates your spinal muscles. As you breathe more and more deeply between your hips and your ribcage, feel your waistline again.

▷ Straighten one leg along the floor. Bring the arm on the same side over your head and stretch it along the floor behind you. The whole of this side of your body should feel stretched and open. As you breathe in, flex your foot and stretch your arm, extending from heel to fingertips. Stretch more as you breathe out. Release and relax. Repeat several times, then change sides and repeat with the other leg and arm. You can also stretch diagonally, extending the opposite arm and leg first one way and then the other, and breathing in the same way.

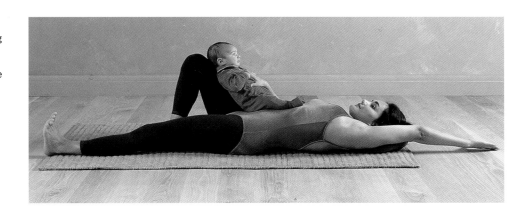

10 Namaste

The pressure of the hands held together in this Indian greeting allows you to breathe more deeply in your upper and middle back. At the same time, you build up inner strength in your open heart area.

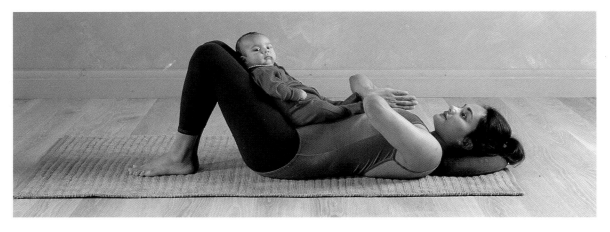

◁ Lying down with your knees bent, join your palms together in front of your heart, in the prayer position. Inhale and press on your palms as you breathe out slowly. Feel the upper back and shoulder muscles strengthening and the front of the chest lifting. At the end of the practice, relax and greet the moment as it is.

Regaining strength and stamina

As you practise the stretches that follow, use Reverse Breathing (1), which will help you stay relaxed and to stretch further. If any area feels tight or tense, breathe out into it to relax it before continuing. Start your stretch from the lower back or pelvis – that is where strength enters, with the breath in. Keep your body relaxed so that you experience the flow of breath while you are stretching.

11 For leg and abdominal muscles

Lie on the floor, reclining against a beanbag or other support. Make sure that your lower back is well supported and your shoulders and neck can stay relaxed. This is a flowing movement in which your legs alternately extend and bend with a relaxed stretch, toning the whole abdomen. If you are able to stretch your legs completely without tensing your abdominal muscles at this stage, you can do so.

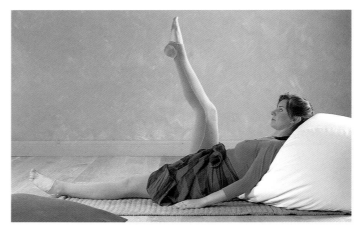

◁ **1** Inhale as you extend your relaxed leg up.

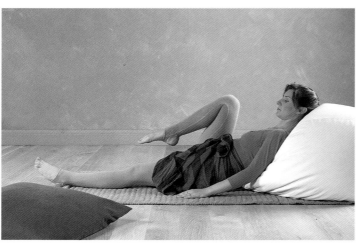

△ **2** Then bend your knee.

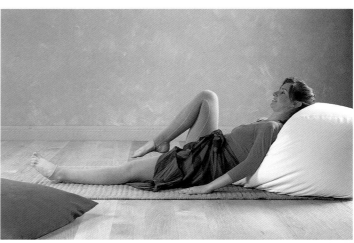

△ **3** Exhale slowly as you extend your leg towards the floor. Extend your leg up again as you inhale and enjoy a smooth circle of movement and breath.

12 For abdominal and pelvic floor muscles, lying down

Practise this exercise as often as you can. Lie on the floor with your legs propped up on a bean-bag or other support.

▷ Bend one knee towards your chest and clasp both hands around your shin. As you breathe out, press your knee to your chest while you also pull your navel up and back towards your spine. This makes your chest widen at the back and lift at the front. Release the pull on your leg before you breathe in again. Repeat a few times, then change leg.

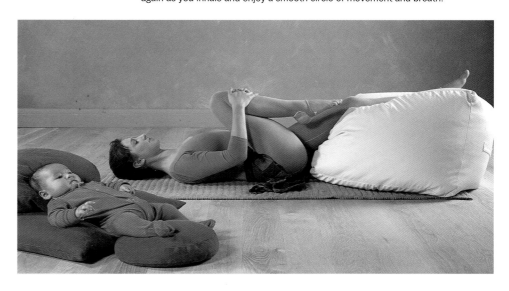

13 For abdominal and pelvic floor muscles, sitting

Sit on a cushion on a firm chair. If you have a Caesarean scar, place a large, soft cushion on your lap to protect your abdomen. Keep your back very straight and your waist against the chair back.

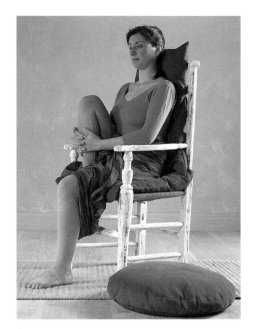

△ Pull your knee to your chest, pressing your foot on the chair. Use Reverse Breathing (1) pulling your knee towards the chest on the breath out. Repeat several times on each side. Keep your face soft and your neck relaxed.

14 For upper back muscles, lying down

Lie on the floor with your legs on a beanbag or a pile of cushions for similar support. Make sure your lower back is comfortable on the floor; if it is not, raise it with a pillow. Relax both your lower back and your legs.

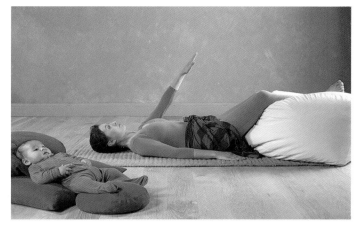

◁ **1** Raise one arm as you breathe in. Stretch it up and then behind your head as you breathe out slowly. Flop the arm back to your side at the end of your out-breath.

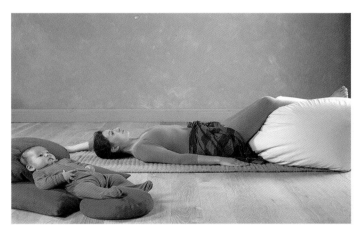

◁ **2** Repeat with your other arm. After a few rounds, work with both arms together. Make sure you keep the back of your waist in contact with the floor throughout, even if you cannot reach the floor behind you with your arms.

15 Wall stretch

Many new mothers find that the weight of their enlarged breasts makes their upper back droop and ache. If you feel like this, the "wall stretch" will help you extend your spine and use deep abdominal breathing to tone and open your back muscles. This stretch also helps prevent mastitis as the overall circulation in the breasts is improved.

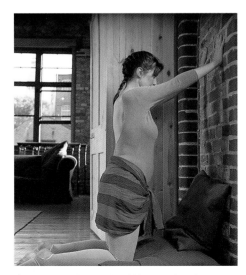

△ **1** With your knees hip-width apart, kneel on a cushion in front of a wall so that when your hands are flat on the wall, your spine is straight.

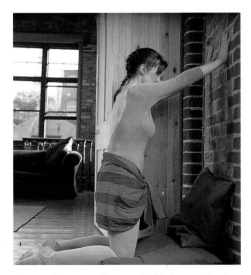

△ **2** Keeping your tailbone tucked in, let your hands slide down the wall very slowly while you breathe as deeply as possible.

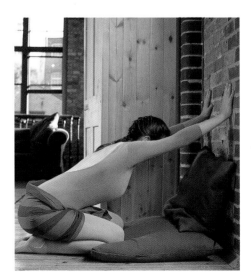

△ **3** Feel your whole spine stretch as you sit on your heels. Continue to elongate your spine for a few breaths. Repeat for a few rounds, or rest.

Spinal stretch

After extending your spine on the floor in the lying down exercises, sitting postures practised on a chair enable you to stretch further and strengthen your lower back from the base of the spine. Sitting upright will also help you to practise Reverse Breathing (1) and pelvic floor lifts more intensely against gravity, as you are working.

16 "Sun wheel" stretch

Sit on an upright chair with your spine erect and feet planted firmly on the floor. Pull your spine upwards from its base to the crown of your head. Keep your neck long and your shoulders down and relaxed.

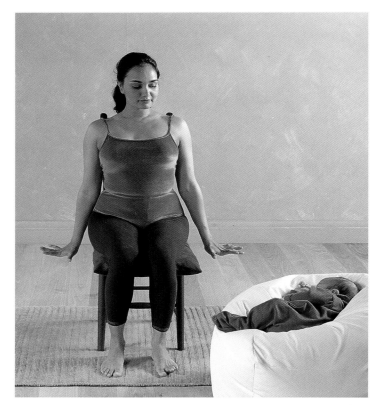

▷ **1** Breathe in. With your out-breath, push your palms down towards the floor, fingers facing out to the sides and wrists bent back in line with your spine. Your shoulder blades draw closer together and your chest expands. Push as if you were moving air currents away from you on the out-breath.

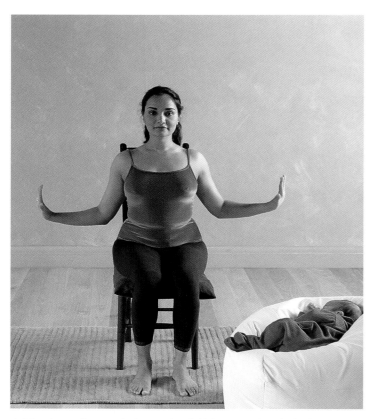

△ **2** Bend your elbows and raise your hands higher as you breathe in, then repeat the downward movement, pushing more on the out-breath.

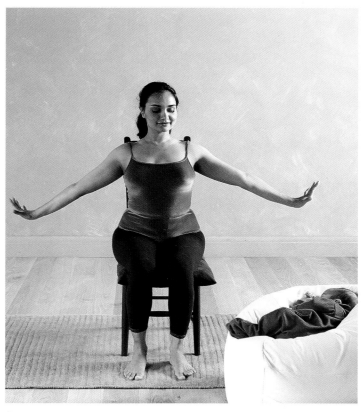

△ **3** Next time you breathe out, push your palms out to your sides at chest level. Keep a flowing movement, breathing in and out.

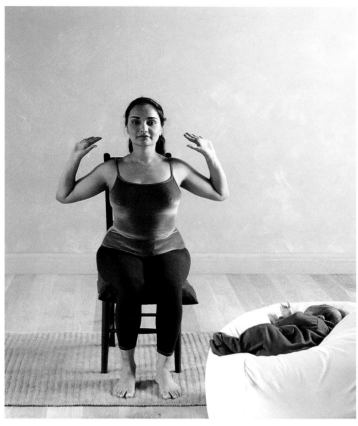

△ **4** As you breathe in your hands are now above your shoulders, opening your upper back and stretching your chest and arm muscles.

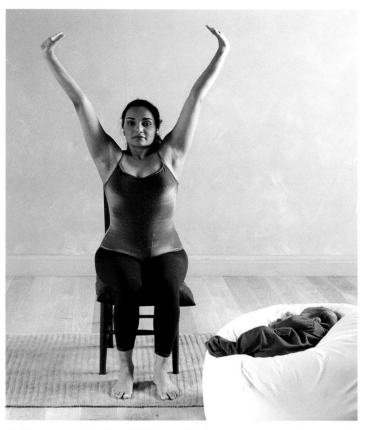

△ **5** Turn your hands out and lift higher and further on your out breath, opening the rib cage. Enjoy your full span, stretching to your fingertips.

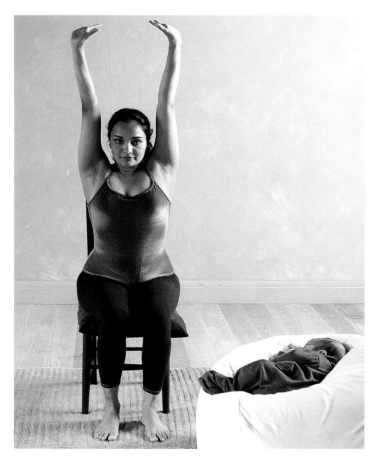

△ **6** On the next round, lift your arms straight up above your head, stretching more as you breathe in. Start your downward wheel by reversing the steps, breathing in your own rhythm with a slow movement.

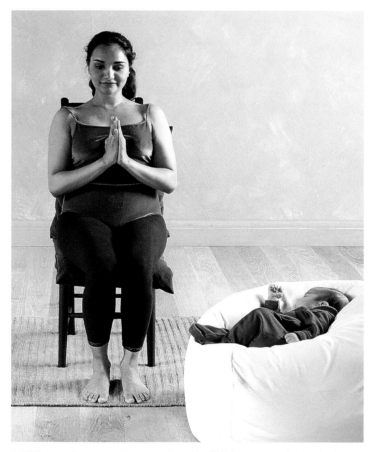

△ **7** When you have completed your "sun wheel", bring your hands together into a seated Namaste position. Press the palms together and breathe quietly, enjoying the effects of this sequence on your whole back.

Gentle twists and bends sitting on a chair

Twisting movements are central to yoga. They are powerful toners, firming the body from inside out in the abdomen and around the waist. Practised gently to begin with after giving birth, twists and their counterparts, forward bends, are very effective means to help new mothers "close" their body again after opening it to grow their babies and give birth.

Yoga twists start from the base of the spine, involving the lumbar area and then progressively the whole back. They stimulate the functioning of all the organs, as the leverage helps you breathe more intensely in the abdomen and chest together. It is usual to twist to the right first, then to the left, as this sequence follows the line of flow in the large intestine. In sitting twists, make

sure you keep the spine stretched up as you twist, from the lower back to the shoulders. The head follows rather than leads this upward slow movement which you expand with your breathing. Twisting is always done on the out breath, and with each out breath, you twist a little further. Today's limit will seem easy after only a week's practice, but never force, just let the extension come.

17 Simple twist on chair
The first twist can be practised soon after giving birth to regain your awareness of your waist. It also opens the chest which helps when you start feeding.

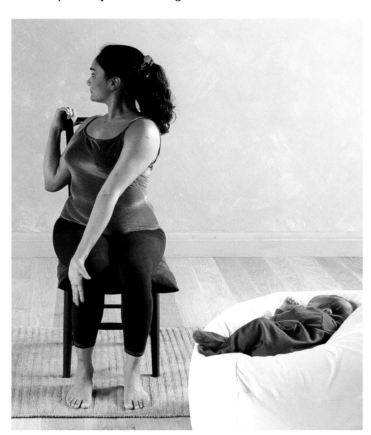

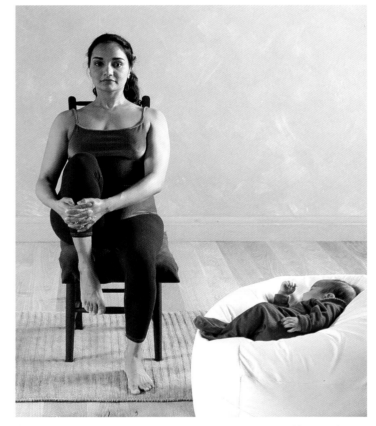

△ **1** Allow your right arm to hang down loosely by your side. Place the back of your left hand against the outside of your right thigh. This hand is your lever: press it against your thigh to help you to twist to the right. As you breathe out, start the twist at the base of the spine and continue it all the way up, so that your neck and face turn last, and you are looking over your right shoulder. Release the twist a little as you breathe in, then increase it as you breathe out again. You can make this simple twist stronger by holding the back of your chair with your right hand. You now have two levers to help you, pushing away from your left hand and pulling towards your right hand. Come back slowly, to face front, as you breathe in.

△ **2** When you have finished, bend your right knee and pull your shin towards your chest as you breathe out. Then twist and bend to the left side. Repeat all these twisting movements to the left.

18 Circling one arm

This is a gentle stretching twist that counters the tension of feeding and stretches the spine. Do it often.

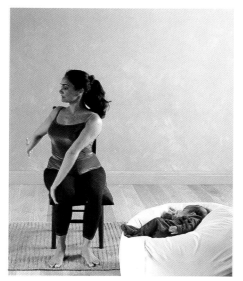

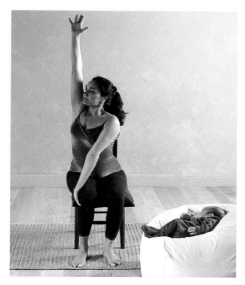

△ **1** Sit upright on your chair, with the back of your left hand outside your right thigh. Stretch out your right arm behind you.

△ **2** Breathing deeply, make a slow circling movement with the extended arm. Repeat on the other side. Then, use your right hand as the lever as you twist to the left and circle your left arm.

19 Crossing your legs

This twist allows a long diagonal stretch that is invigorating.

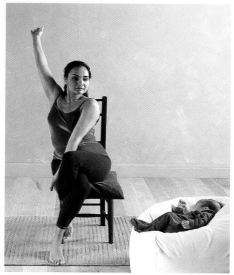

△ Cross your left leg over your right knee and – if you can – tuck your toes behind your right calf. Use your left hand as the lever, pressing it against the outside of your right thigh. Twist to the right, circling your right arm in a wide sweep up in front and down behind you, breathing deeply. Repeat on the other side.

20 Forward bend (1)

Bending forward after giving birth may feel slightly uncomfortable at first. You have not been able to bend for a long time, and now bending may remind you that your body has changed. Trust that yoga will help you tone your body in depth day by day. If you have had a Caesarian section, place a pillow on your lap before bending forward.

▷ When you have finished the twisting movements, relax completely. Extend your right foot along the floor and ease your lower back by flopping forward, breathing out. Extend your arms to your shins, ankles or, if you can, to your toes. Repeat with the left foot, and then extend both feet, breathing deeply with long, slow, relaxing breaths out.

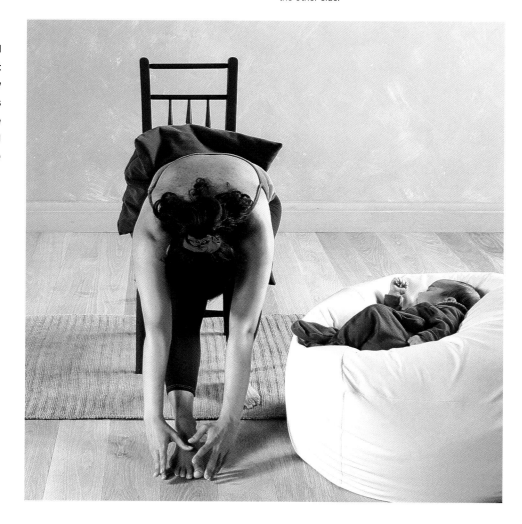

Standing twists with a chair

The arm movements for this sequence are the same as for the twists sitting on a chair, but this time you should stand in front of the chair with your right foot placed firmly upon the seat. Make sure that the chair is the correct height for your knee to be bent at a right angle with your standing leg straight. There are two twists: "open" and "closed".

Only practise the "closed" twist when you are comfortable with the full extension of the "open" twist. In standing twists, the whole torso turns and extends following the circling of the arm. The leverage of the arms helps you to draw in your pelvic floor muscles as you twist.

21 Open twist

In this twist, one arm is used as a lever on the inside of the same leg to allow the trunk to open and rotate.

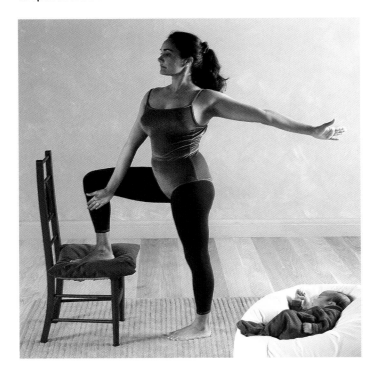

◁ Place one foot on the chair with the back of your hand acting as a lever on the inside of your thigh. Twist away from the raised leg and circle your other arm. Repeat on the other side. Breathe deeply as you circle your arms, always using the out-breath to twist further with the stretch.

22 Closed twist (1)

In this twist, one arm is used as a lever on the outside of the opposite leg to bring about a more intense rotation at the base of the spine. As the trunk turns, the kidneys and abdominal organs are activated and exercised.

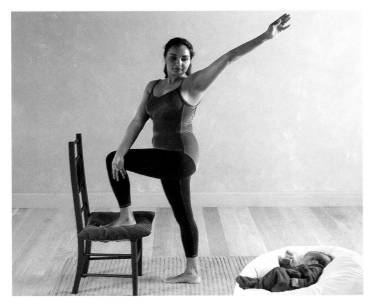

△ Place one foot on the chair with your opposite hand as a lever on the outside of your thigh, then twist towards the raised leg and circle your free arm. Repeat on the other side. Keep your chest very open.

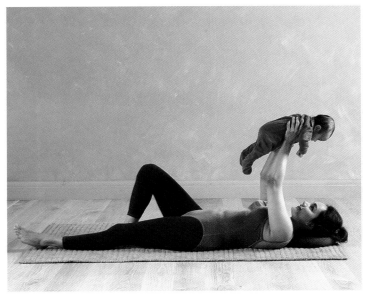

△ After doing standing twists it is a good idea to lie down with one or both knees bent for a short rest. It will soon be playtime!

Relieving tension in the back

The floor twist can be practised either as a gentler completion of a sequence of sitting and standing twists, or just on its own to relieve tension in the back whenever you need it. Sometimes this may be several times a day... If you have not had time to do a full yoga sequence, the lying down twist is a good exercise to do before going into a deep relaxation.

23 Floor twist

Before doing the twist on the floor, ease your lower back by bending your knees and rolling gently on the small of your back.

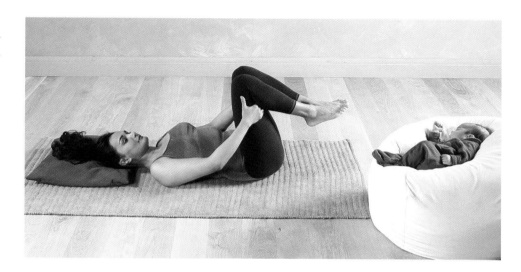

▷ **1** Place your hands at the back of your thighs, just below your knees. Practise Reverse Breathing (1), breathing in and pulling the perineum up. Draw your knees closer to your chest, breathing out as you pull your waist back and open the back. Repeat a few times to loosen up your lower and middle back.

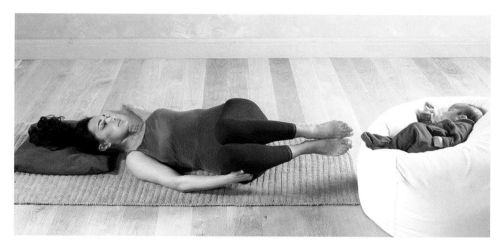

◁ **2** Extend your left arm along the floor. Feel the upper back widening and the shoulder relaxing. Gravity is your lever here – the relaxed weight of your upper body and left arm pin you to the floor. Breathe in and, on the out-breath, drop your bent legs to the right with your right hand supporting their weight. If you are flexible enough, your legs and feet may come to rest on the floor. If so, leave them there for a few breaths. To make the twist stronger, you can also turn your head towards your extended arm.

▷ **3** Breathe in to bring your legs back to the starting position over your chest, using your right hand to help lift their weight. Repeat the movement to the left and continue several times on each side. Relax with your knees bent to finish.

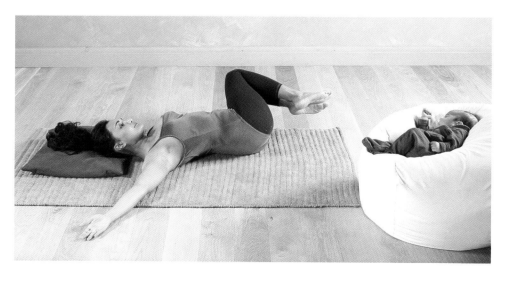

Basic kneeling sequence

These movements strengthen and relax the whole body. They will give you a good workout, improving flexibility and lifting your spirits. The movements should be learnt separately, then practised as a routine that flows with the rhythm of your natural breathing. If you have done yoga before, you may recognize a kneeling version of the "sun salute". In this version, you remain close to the floor to avoid straining your abdominal muscles, which are not yet ready for the full sequence. The exercises are also complete in themselves and can be practised separately. Always relax at the end of the kneeling sun salute. You can return to the Swan Pose and rest or lie in Shavasana (27). Try to get into the habit of relaxing, even for a minute, after completing every sequence.

24 Swan pose

In this relaxing pose, the stretched arms help you breathe more deeply in the middle and lower back. This can be very soothing.

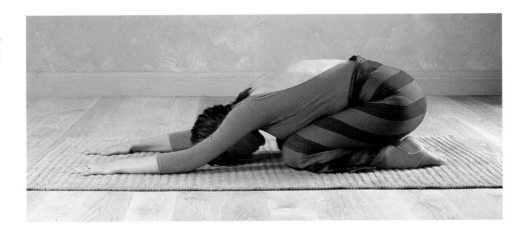

▷ **1** Relax and stretch in this pose, sitting on your heels. Extend your fingers forward for maximum stretch. Press on your hands when you exhale.

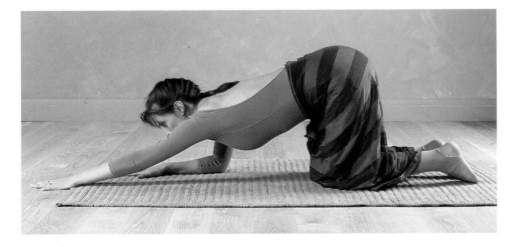

◁ **2** Bending your right arm so that your forearm can rest on the floor, stretch your left arm forward as far as you can, extending your fingers. At the same time, allow your spine to extend backwards, breathing into the stretch which reaches from your hand to the base of the spine. Change sides and repeat.

▷ **3** Bend your elbow to open your chest fully. Rotate the shoulder, breathing into the circular movement of your bent arm. Replace your forearm on the floor and work the other side. Change sides and repeat. Rest afterwards with your head and arms down, as before, if you feel tired.

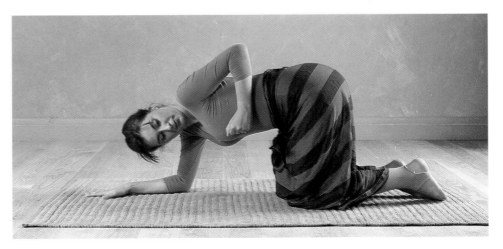

25 Cat pose

This is an easy way to stretch your spine. In a steady "on all fours" position, alternate an upward and downward circling of the back together with an inhalation and an exhalation.

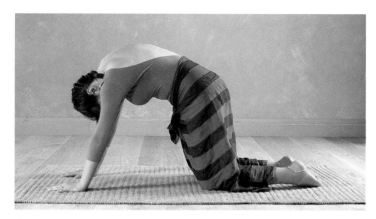

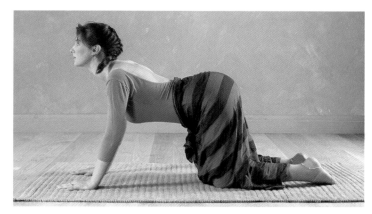

△ **1** Come on to all fours, with your back flat. Your knees should be hip-width apart: the hip directly over the knee and the shoulder over the wrist. Spread your fingers for good support. Breathing in, arch your spine and tuck your head in.

△ **2** Breathing out, flatten your back at the waist and look up. Repeat. If you wish, you can create a flowing movement, bending your arms to roll back and forth in the stretch.

26 Leg stretches

Lower backache is common in the weeks after giving birth. Leg stretches can both prevent and ease tension, particularly around the sciatic nerve.

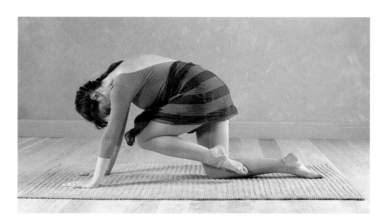

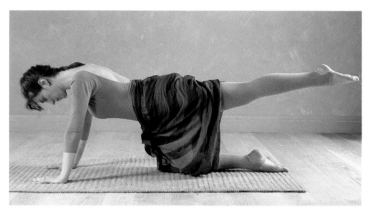

△ **1** Starting in the Cat Pose, above, breathe in and bring one bent knee forward towards your face, keeping the calf muscle and foot relaxed.

△ **2** Breathing out, stretch that leg out behind you (keeping it relaxed). Your body, from crown to heel, stretches in a straight line. Extend your out-breath as much as possible.

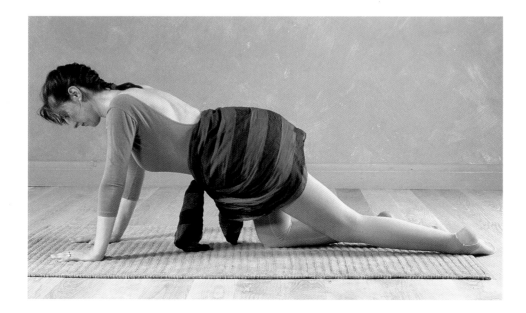

◁ **3** Turn your extended foot inwards and drop it on the floor, relaxing your leg and trailing it limply, allowing the hip to drop. From this position, bring your bent knee forward again to repeat the three steps several times. Then change legs.

Healing relaxation from six weeks

This relaxation is not just to recover from your exertions after a yoga session or to rest after a disturbed night. It is for healing, and for integrating the whole experience of pregnancy and childbirth into your life.

The period of six weeks after giving birth is known as "postpartum". The six-week point signals the ending of one phase and the start of another, as you cease to be a "new" mother and become instead a mother. As you pass from one stage to the next it is important to avoid taking any unnecessary physical or emotional baggage with you. You want to move on feeling healed and whole, ready to enjoy your baby.

Six weeks is about the average time it takes to recover from giving birth. For you it may be shorter or longer – you will know when you have reached this dividing line. But even when the birth experience is many months behind you it is still a good idea to do this focused relaxation from time to time. It helps you to assess how well you are moving on into the flow of your life, and free remaining areas of tension.

conscious surrender

This pose seems very simple, but it involves considerable body awareness, which only comes with practice. Breathe the tension away, then move on to visualizing your happy scene in which you are experiencing total well-being.

From that contented space, look at any unhappy feelings that sometimes afflict you. Be brave and honest with yourself. Acknowledge your own feelings of tiredness and low spirits. Accept them as part of how your life is, and how you are.

We are all just as we are. Judgment and perfectionist standards (your own or anyone else's) have no place here. Simply soothe and care for yourself, just as you would for a dear friend who came to you for loving support. Be your own dearest and most reliable friend – and learn to accept help from this source of inner strength.

You may become aware of other feelings, too. Unacknowledged anger is common: anger at the disruption to your life since your baby was born, anger at feeling disorganized, anger at other people, anger at having to put aside your own interests. These are just a few of the issues that may come up. You may also experience feelings of sadness: grief for the time before you had responsibilities, or for

"As I sit quietly with you my child, I ask that I be made a strong and loving parent. May your life always be filled with light."

▽ **As you quieten the body and the mind in stillness, allow this conscious relaxation to free you from fluctuating emotions.**

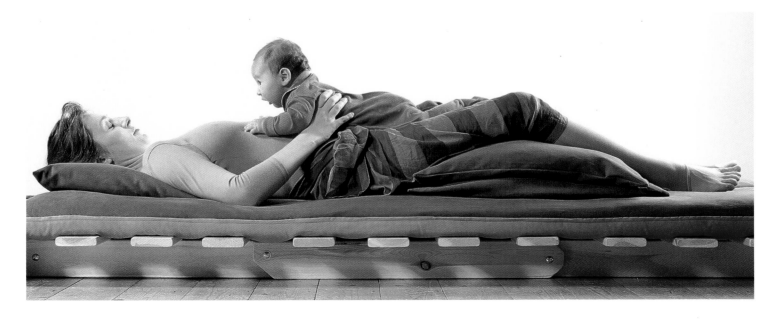

the loss of your own childhood, or for those golden days when you never seemed to run out of energy.

Mixed emotions are normal at this stage, around six weeks after the birth. They may come as the result of changes in lifestyle, or hormonal changes as your body returns to its pre-pregnant state, or a mixture of both. The first step in dealing with any such feelings is to admit that you feel them. Then tell your "inner friend" all about your sad or angry feelings and ask for understanding, support and healing. These are already there for you – you have only to ask. Emotional burdens can be lifted from you simply by acknowledging them and sharing them with that "inner friend" who loves you and whom you know you can trust. Be humble and true to yourself as you do this.

Having accepted and then released your negative feelings, you can fully experience and share all your feelings of love and joy. Take time to allow them to surface. Tell your baby of your great love, and tell the other members of your family that you love them, too. Draw them all together into the circle of your love. Recognize and be grateful for the deep joy that is welling up within you and radiating outwards to everyone around you. Breathe gently in and out of your heart space for a few moments.

When you are ready, let the vision fade away. Become aware of your breathing and expand it slowly until you are back in focus. Then move your fingers and toes. Finally, s-t-r-e-t-c-h and yawn before starting to sit up. Remember that the deeper your state of relaxation, the more important it is to come out of it slowly.

27 Shavasana

Refer back to the basic relaxation technique, although by now it should be second nature to you. Your position should be a comfortable one that you can maintain without moving. Shavasana, or the Corpse Pose, is a classic yoga relaxation pose. Once you are settled and comfortable, avoid any further movements. Close your eyes and just let go. Scan your body from the inside and, wherever you find any tension, melt it away and nurture that space. Do the same with any images or emotions that arise, connected with your birthing experience.

To come out of the pose, expand your breath gently but steadily, until you feel drawn to open your eyes effortlessly. Feel your body come back into focus. Then stretch before you sit up. Relaxation is progressive – each time you practise, it helps you to go deeper next time.

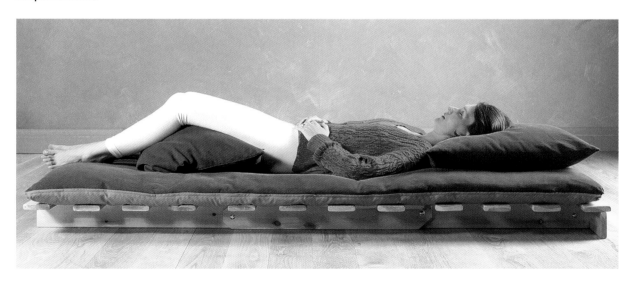

◁ Lie down comfortably, at a time when you can expect to be undisturbed for at least ten minutes – hopefully longer.

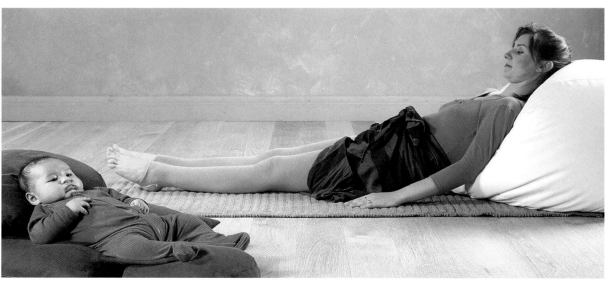

◁ If it is more comfortable, you can have your head and shoulders supported by a beanbag or pillow. Relaxation can be practised in bed when you need it.

Pulling up

Realigning the spine after giving birth may take time and dedication. But persevere because it is a very important process which lays the foundation for your future well-being as it may determine your long term posture. "Standing tall" refers not only to having a straight back, but also to using your pelvic floor, abdominal muscles and lower back muscles to hold your pelvis in perfect alignment with your spine. Then stretching becomes truly beneficial… You will look and feel amazing.

28 Tadasana: standing tall

This is a classic yoga pose and is used as a starting position for many others. With a vertical support, use your awareness in this pose to realign the spine after pregnancy. You can line yourself up against a wall or the edge of a door, to get into the correct position, and then take a step away without losing your "line". Reverse Breathing (1) will greatly assist you.

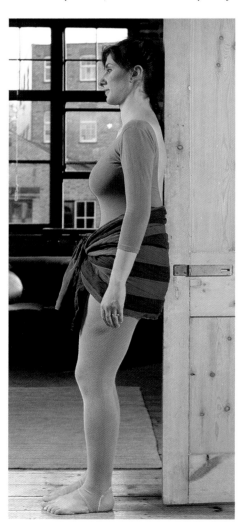

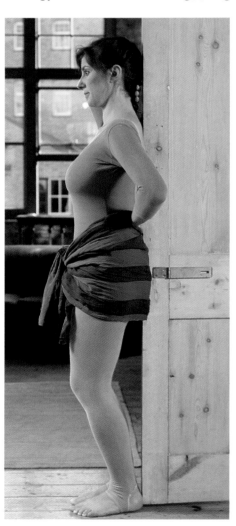

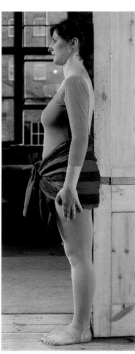

◁ **3** After breathing in position 2 for a while, straighten your legs again and stand tall against the door. Check your best position today. Breathe deeply, feeling your alignment. Every day will be different.

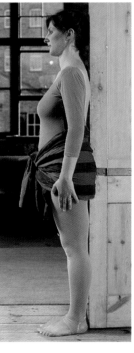

◁ **4** After doing this you can also practise standing on one leg and circling the other foot inwards and outward, exercising your ankles and feet arches.

△ **1** With your knees loosely bent and your feet a foot's length away from the door or wall, line up your spine all along its length. Pull up the lower abdominal muscles as you breathe in. Bring the waist back and open the chest as you breathe out. Draw your chin and neck back.

△ **2** Bring your heels close to the door. With your hands, explore the hollow behind your waist. Bend your knees slightly, more if you have done yoga before, to align your spine. Remove your hands. Use Reverse Breathing (1), to strengthen your back muscles, drawing in your pelvic floor muscles – deep as you inhale and further as you exhale.

Protecting your lower back

Babies soon get heavy and it is easy to strain yourself when lifting and carrying them around, particularly in seats and carriers.

Remember that your abdominal muscles are likely to be overstretched from giving birth, so they cannot do their normal job of protecting your lower back. Compensate for any weakness by making the best use of your leg muscles and upper back.

29 Standing up, holding your baby

Your baby may join you on the floor while you practise your yoga, change a nappy, or breastfeed between sequences. Several times a day, practise getting up from the floor, and getting down, holding your baby with your back strong and straight. You will soon develop strength and poise.

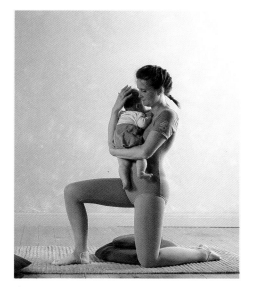

△ **1** Kneel, then rise on to one knee, using your arms and upper back to support the baby's weight.

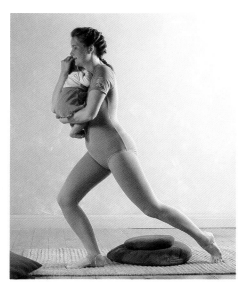

△ **2** Take your weight on to your front leg, turning the toes of your back foot under, and rise.

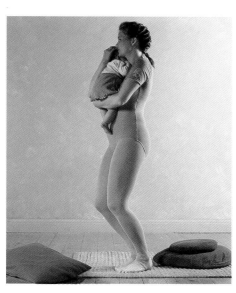

△ **3** Straighten your knees only after your spine is erect and you feel balanced.

30 Bathing your baby

It is common for new mothers to strain their backs while bathing their babies. Yoga helps you to develop an awareness of the way in which you reach forward and can lift your baby most easily.

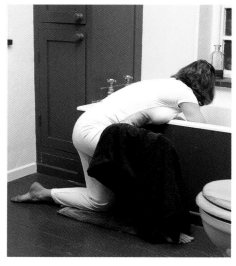

△ **1** Kneel on one knee, as close to the bath as possible, with a towel at the ready.

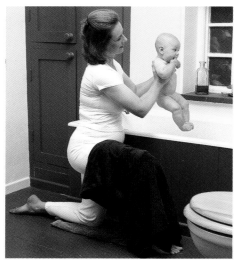

△ **2** Take a deep in-breath as you lift your baby, completing the lift on an out-breath.

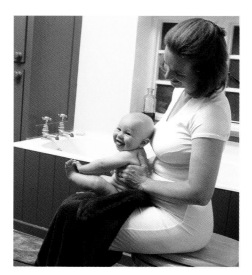

△ **3** Sit upright as you dry the baby.

Yoga every day

Once the basic techniques in this section have become really familiar to you, any spare time can be used for yoga. Here are some suggestions, and you will soon discover other ideas yourself. Be creative! Remember to use Reverse Breathing (1), and to practise your deep relaxation daily. Always rest for a few moments after yoga breathing and stretching.

yoga breathing

Get into the habit of using Reverse Breathing (1) at any time of the day or night, whatever position you happen to be in. Every breath in draws the energy of life – of vitality and healing – into the abdominal cavity to strengthen and tone the stretched muscles of the perineum and abdomen.

Every long breath out allows the energy of love – of openness and relationship – to lift the chest and the spirits and to open the upper back and the heart space. As these two aspects of universal energy blend, and flow up the spine to the crown of the head, you feel a light energy in and around you. Your mind becomes focused, clear and serene and your posture upright and confident.

The benefits seem purely physical at first but, as you continue to practise, you will find that deep and beneficial changes occur; you you are being healed at many levels. This is the magic of yoga.

relaxation

This is an essential part of any yoga session. Always include a resting position after every sequence and a relaxation at the end of your session. Rest is healing and deep relaxation will replace lost sleep. Alternate Nostril Breathing (2) is a quick and effective way to centre yourself at any time, and a good way to begin each yoga session.

good posture

Use Reverse Breathing (1) to help draw yourself upright every time you feel that you are drooping. Use your upper back and leg muscles to take the strain off your abdominal and lower back muscles.

stretches

Always start your stretches from the lower back. Avoid tensing your legs or arms – stay loose and use your breath to extend further.

31 Minding your posture in the kitchen

While you are waiting for the kettle to boil, or for something to finish cooking, you can realign your posture and practise Reverse Breathing (1) to tone your abdominal muscles in depth from the pelvic floor.

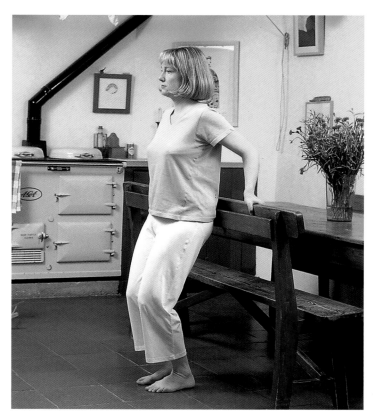

△ **1** Strengthen your thigh muscles by bending your knees. You can support yourself by bending your elbows behind you and leaning on a table or chair back.

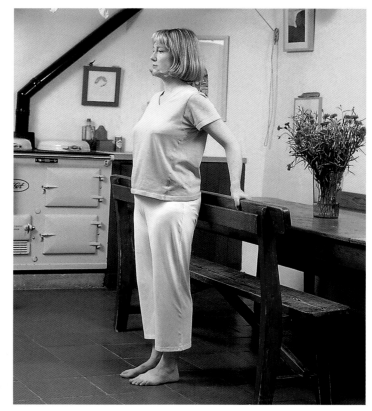

△ **2** Bend and straighten your knees, keeping your spine erect and your chest open. As you stand up, inhale and lift, exhaling as you bend.

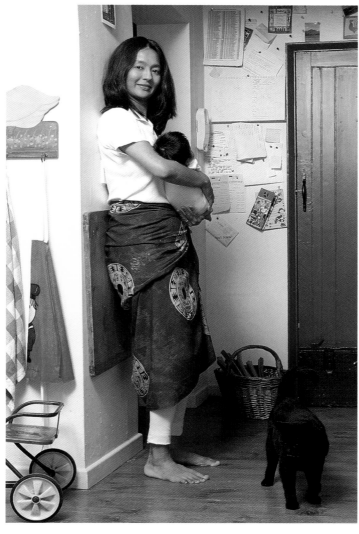

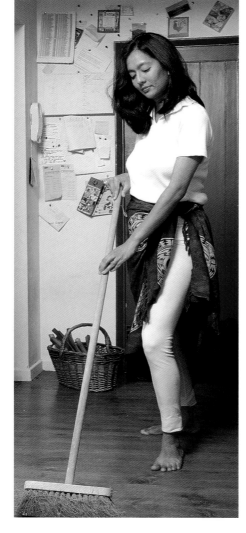

◁ You can lean against a wall in any spare moment, drawing up your spine and keeping it in contact with the wall.

▷ Remember your posture when doing housework. Aim to keep your knees bent and your spine erect. Bend your knees before leaning forward or lifting anything.

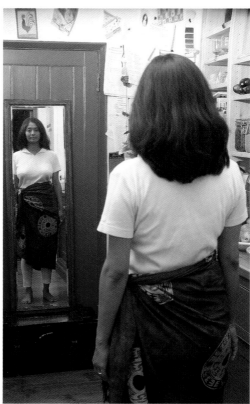

△ Stand in front of a long mirror from time to time to check your progress.

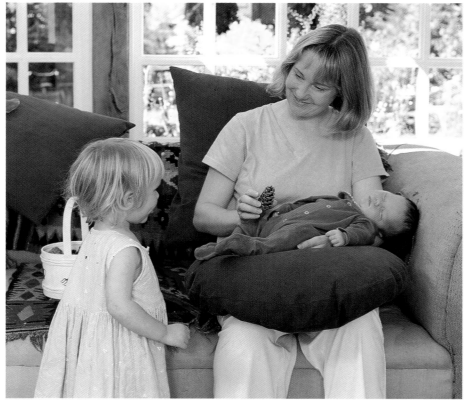

△ Stop, relax and enjoy life whenever you can – it is time well spent, time that will not return. Babies grow very quickly and the days rush by.

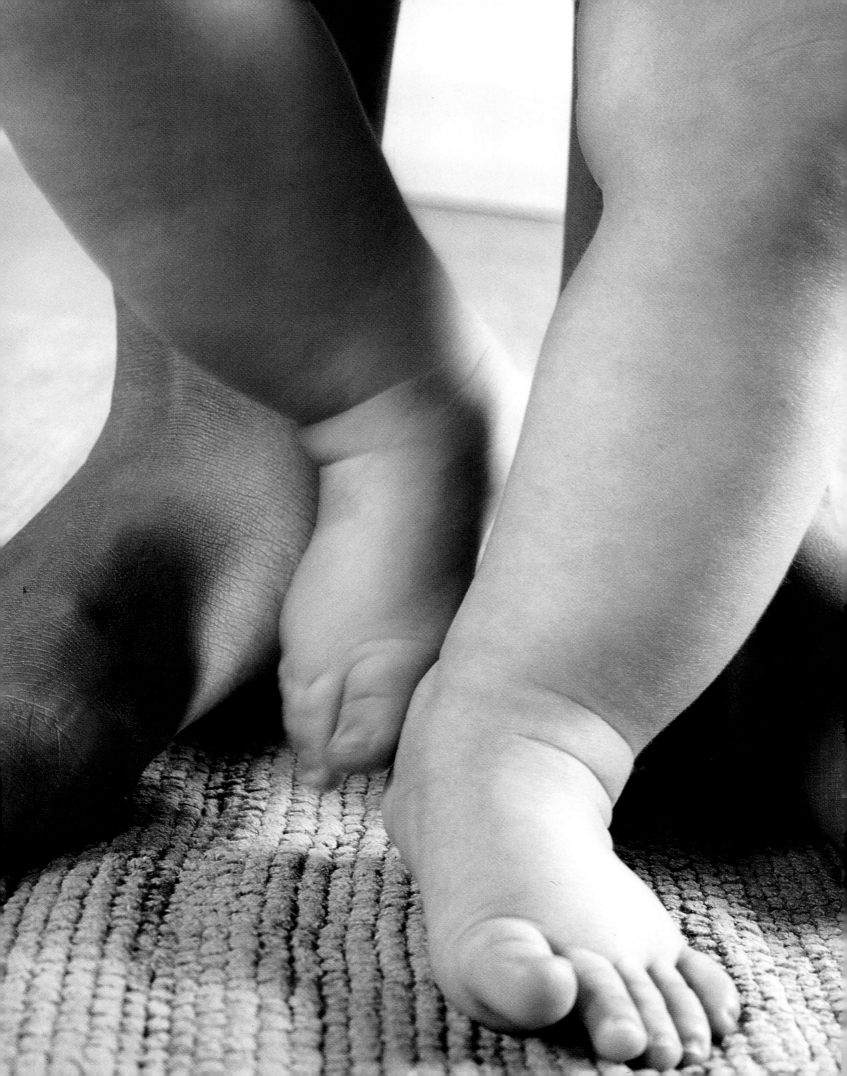

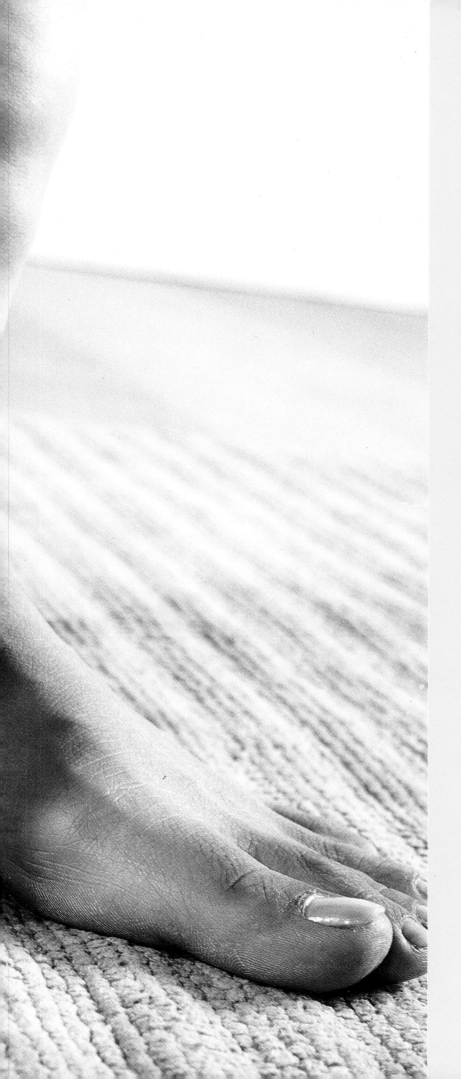

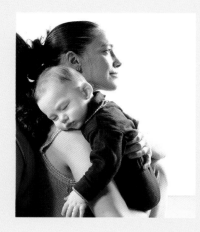

gentle
progression

Rest, more rest and relaxation come before

exercise. Each yoga posture becomes a

therapy in itself that stimulates but also

calms you, energizes but also nurtures you

in a comfortable, effortless way. Take time

to watch your body rhythms and your

feelings as you stretch more without ever

straining, letting your breathing guide you.

Six to twelve weeks after birth

The next set of exercises is more demanding, and should provide just what you need from six weeks to twelve weeks after giving birth. You will have had your postnatal check-up and are now probably ready to move on to some more classic yoga.

Everyone is different, however, and you should check your progress before moving on. You may have practised less than you would have liked over the last six weeks. You may feel that you still need to stick with the earlier routines for a while longer, for any number of reasons.

One reason may be that you have only just acquired this book! If this is the case, it is essential first to familiarize yourself very thoroughly with the basics of Reverse Breathing (1), relaxation and stretching.

The yoga techniques in this chapter form the foundation for ongoing physical, emotional and mental well-being. One of the ancient yoga texts emphasizes that, "In yoga no effort, however small, is ever wasted." However advanced you may become in your yoga practice, you should still make time to stretch and relax daily, and to be always conscious of your breathing and your posture. It takes only a minute to

"Nothing prepared me for the highs and the lows, the challenges, the defeats and the victories. It took weeks to become a mother and still be who I am."

practise a few reverse breaths, pulling yourself up from the perineum to the crown and opening your chest and your heart space. Get into the habit of doing this several times every day, wherever you happen to be.

The routines in this section will help you to consolidate your pelvic strength and the realignment of your spine. Some more yoga "asanas" (poses) will be introduced, as well as vigorous limbering sequences that really get the energy flowing. You will continue to breathe deeply and to make relaxation your priority – this is an essential ingredient

within every movement as well as during your rest afterwards.

Sometimes you may have only a few moments to spare. If your baby needs your attention when you are in the middle of a routine, go back to your starting position and take a deep breath out to relax. Then smile, as you go to greet your baby.

▽ **As you get ready for more active yoga, remember that relaxation is the foundation for renewing your strength and stamina from within. Keep using the relaxations from the first section.**

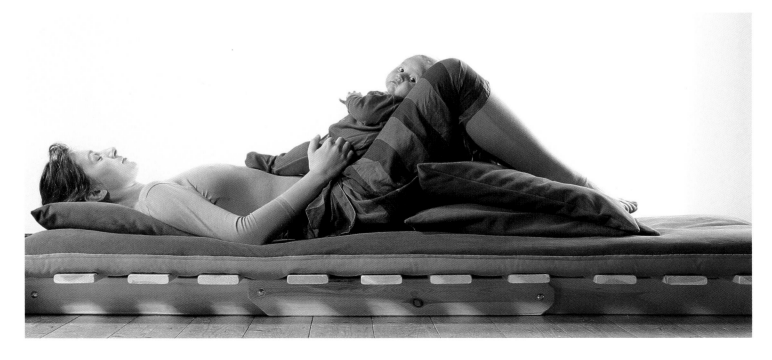

More advanced reverse breathing

The following positions – described in order of difficulty – allow you to get a really good "grip" on your pelvic floor muscles as you breathe in and out. You are now using the buttock muscles too. After pregnancy, it may be unfamiliar to you. First become aware of the power of your buttock muscles, tightening them and then releasing them, before practising the exercises on this page.

32 Standing against the wall

Tightening your buttock muscles intensifies the "pulling up" that you practised in Tadasana (28).

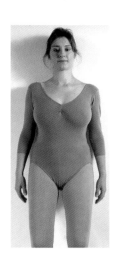

◁ **1** Stand with your heels a short distance away from a wall. Then place your spine against the wall, keeping your knees bent. Tightening your buttocks, breathe in and pull the pelvic floor up. Hold the grip as you breathe out, then relax all the muscles. Repeat several times.

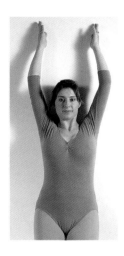

◁ **2** For a more extreme posture, raise your arms against the wall as you breathe in and repeat the exercise several times.

33 Raising the hips

Tightening your buttock muscles as well as practising Reverse Breathing (1) makes this apparently easy raising of the hips from the floor a very powerful toner.

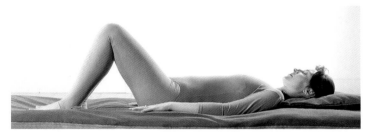

△ **1** Lie on the floor with your knees bent and feet flat on the floor, hip-width apart. Lengthen the back of your neck and keep your chin tucked in throughout. Place your arms alongside your body, palms down, to support you.

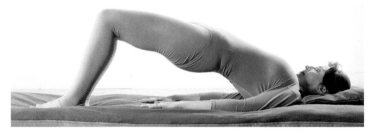

△ **2** As you breathe in, lift your pelvis up from the floor as high as you comfortably can, keeping your inner knees in a straight line. Grip the base of your spine with your buttock muscles and hold as you breathe out. Lift your pelvic floor again as you breathe in again, then relax as you breathe out.

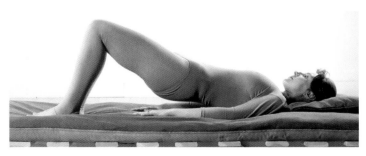

△ **3** On your next in-breath, release the buttock muscles and lower your pelvis slowly to the floor, lengthening your spine as far towards your heels as possible. Repeat several times.

34 Lying prone

This position is one that you won't have been able to achieve for some time whilst pregnant. Now, it offers you a different angle for pelvic floor lifts.

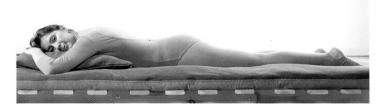

△ Lie on your front with cushions under your breasts and your upper back wide and relaxed, with your elbows bent at eye level and your face turned to one side. Let your feet roll apart. Grip the base of your spine with your buttock muscles. Breathe in and out a few times, then release.

gentle progression

In this chapter, like the last, the yoga poses have been modified to provide you with a gentle progression, and are especially useful for those new to yoga. If you find any of these poses too difficult for now, do not worry, you can simply compose a sequence to suit you from the other poses in this section. Many standing poses can also be practised more easily with your back against

a wall. If you stand a half-foot away from the wall, you can then use it as a support for your back by leaning against it while in the pose.

Some standing poses are described here as rhythmical sequences. Movement that flows with the breath is relaxing, effective and more "yogic" than a stretch in which you try and conform to a pre-set notion of how you should look in a posture. Before

you feel comfortable holding "asanas", the word for classical yoga poses which implies steadiness of body, breath and mind, you can practise at least some of them using movement and rhythm. When you hold a pose, however, the dynamic is created inside your body with breathing. This is what makes yoga poses enjoyable. Whenever you feel tension, come out of it and relax.

35 Dynamic archer pose

As you become stronger day by day, stand tall in Tadasana (28), which is also known as the Mountain Pose, and feel the strong vertical axis between earth and sky.

▷ **1** Stand in Tadasana (28). This is the starting pose for standing postures in yoga.

▷ **2** Jump or walk your feet about 1m/3ft apart. Turn your right foot out, your left foot in. Inhale, raising your arms open to shoulder level without tensing them. Exhale bending your right knee and turning your head right, extending both arms as much as you can. Inhale, straighten your legs, centre your head and turn the left foot out, right foot in. Exhale, stretching to the left. Continue alternating sides in an easy rhythm.

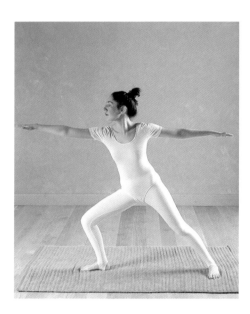

36 "Easy" triangle pose (Trikonasana)

Find an easy rhythm, stretching only as far as you can go without disturbing your relaxed breathing. This sequence combines a stretch (the Archer Pose) (35) and an open twist in the Triangle Pose.

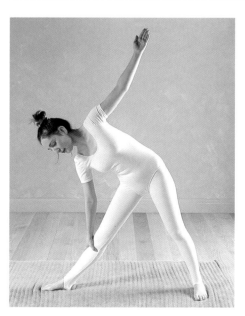

◁ **1** Begin in the Archer Pose, above. With your feet still apart and your arms extended, tilt your trunk to the right. Breathe naturally, letting your right hand slide down your right leg to the point where you feel you cannot go any further down without bending forward. Lift the inner arch of your right foot.

▷ **2** Keeping your weight on the left leg, inhale and stretch from your left heel all the way to the fingertips of your left hand. Look at your left hand and stretch more as you exhale. Come back to centre and repeat on the left side.

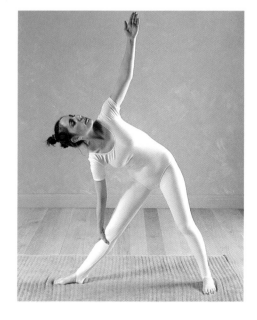

37 "Easy" forward bend

It is pleasant to let gravity stretch your spine while your shoulders, neck and head can relax completely in this forward bend, which also stretches the back of your legs.

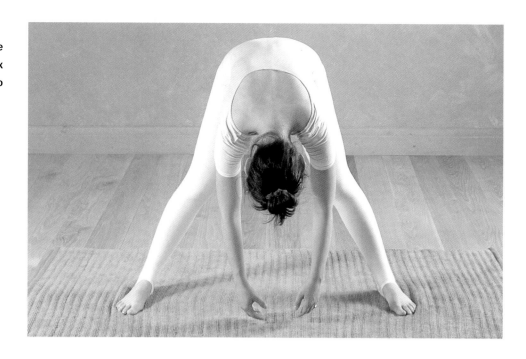

▷ When you have stretched both sides a couple of times, come back to the centre and lower your arms to flop into a gentle forward bend. Relax your neck. You may like to swing your head and shoulders gently from side to side, to ease your lower back. Bend your knees as you breathe in to come up from this pose.

38 "Easy" tree pose (Vrkasana)

Start with a low chair or stool for this pose and graduate to a higher one as you become more confident and flexible. (You may prefer to have your back against a wall to do both this pose, and the Eagle Pose (Garudasana) (39), if your balance is unsteady.)

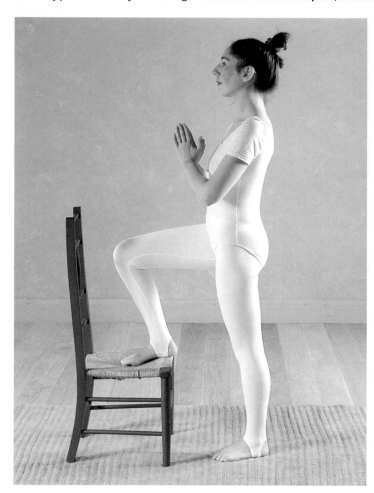

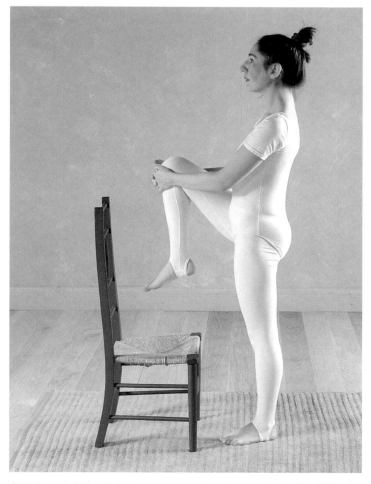

△ **1** Stand in Tadasana (28), facing the chair. Place one foot on the chair and bring your hands into Namaste (10) (the prayer position). Use deep breathing to stretch and align your spine and centre your energies. Hold the pose with your body, breath and mind remaining steady.

△ **2** When you feel ready, bring your knee up towards your chest, with both hands clasped below your knee. Keep steady and balanced, with your spine in line. As you breathe out squeeze your bent leg towards your body and release as you breathe in. Breathing deeply, hold the position for a moment. Release, regain your balance and steadiness, then bend the other knee and repeat.

Movement and rhythm can make yoga postures dynamic, energetic and fun at a time when you spend a great deal of time at home with your baby. The various walks on this page can be done at any time, with or without your baby, whenever you feel like moving your body. Do not forget to breathe and to relax while you stretch!

39 Eagle Pose (Garudasana)

This is another balancing pose, which is very "closing" and excellent for improving concentration. It is easiest to do it quickly, without thinking too much about what goes where! Avoid twisting your spine to achieve the position – it is better to be content with wrapping yourself up more loosely.

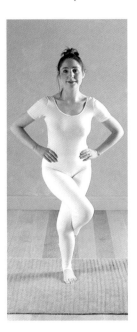

◁ **1** Stand in Tadasana (28) and centre yourself. Rest your hands on the tops of your hips and breathe in. As you breathe out, bend your knees, wrap your right leg around your left leg and – if you can – tuck your right foot behind your left calf. Hold this position, breathing deeply.

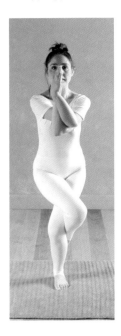

◁ **2** Only when you feel comfortable add the arms. Raise your bent left arm in front of your face and bring your bent right arm around it. Bring your palms together. Sit down with your back erect, as if on an invisible chair, and focus on your fingers, directly in front of your face. With practice you will be able to do both movements together on one breath. Change sides and repeat.

40 Cross-stride walking

This is a dynamic movement to do in any odd moments, or to shake yourself out after the static standing poses. It is the opposite to the way most of us walk, and it takes concentration to co-ordinate the right and left sides. Cross-striding is very good for lifting the spirit, and there are dozens of different movements you can create with different rhythms.

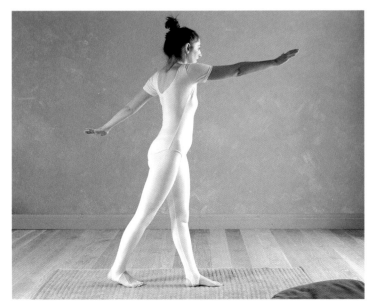

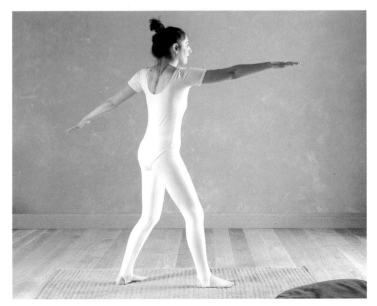

△ **1** Stride briskly with long steps and arms swinging up to shoulder level. Note that your right arm comes forward when your right leg is at the back and your right arm goes back when your right leg comes forward.

△ **2** Now change to cross-stride walking, bringing your right arm and leg forward together, then your left arm and leg.

41 Cross-stride prancing

You can do this using your baby as a "weight", to strengthen your arm muscles and upper back. Grasp your baby firmly with one arm around the chest and the other between the legs so that you can swing him or her vigorously from side to side: your baby might love it. Prance around the room, garden or park with a light step and a light heart.

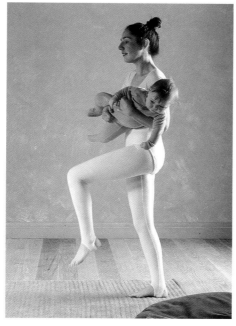

△ **1** Walk in a rhythm first, raising one knee up at a time while you swing your shoulders to the opposite side of the raised knee.

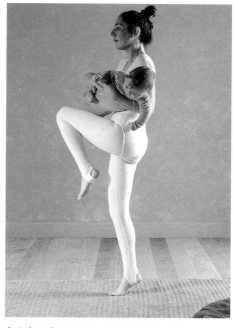

△ **2** Then rise on to your toes, bring your knee even higher and twist even more, before stepping lightly forward and raising the other knee.

42 Walking warrior pose

To prepare for this movement, stand in Tadasana (28) first. The length of your stride will depend on the flexibility of your hips. Get into a flowing, walking rhythm, extending your stride as your hips loosen. Practise without your baby at first, then invite him or her to join you.

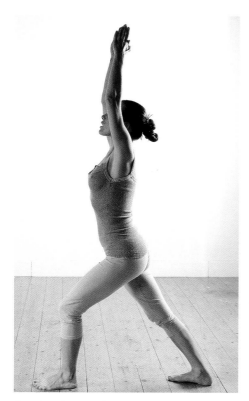

△**1** Take a long step forward. Bend your front knee. Keep your weight on the outside of your back foot and your spine erect. Breathe in and, as you breathe out, raise your arms straight overhead with your palms facing each other. Look up and stretch more as you exhale. Then lower your arms as you bring your back foot forward for your next stretch.

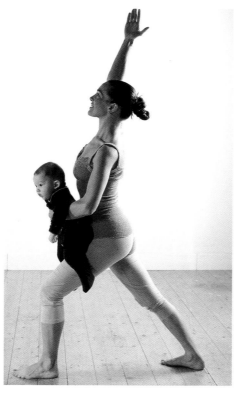

△ **2** Your baby can join in. Rest him or her on your bent leg with one hand supporting, and stretch the other arm overhead.

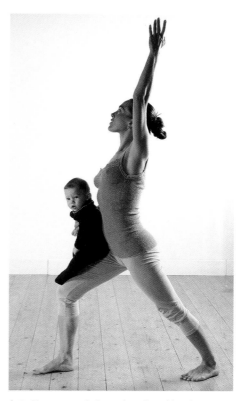

△ **3** Change your baby to the other side when you take your other leg forward.

Kneeling sequence: stretches, bends and twists

Sitting on your knees enables you to lift your lower spine and stretch without straining your lower back and abdominal muscles. Yoga "asanas" in this position straighten your back and make your spine strong and supple. They also tone your thigh muscles in a way that may surprise you at first. They remove fatigue and refresh your whole body with little effort.

43 Vajrasana

This is a classic sitting pose in which you can develop the awareness of your vertical axis – from the pelvic floor to the crown.

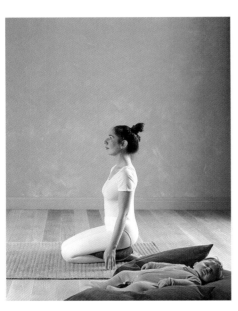

◁ Sit on your heels with your feet stretched out flat behind you and your spine and head erect. You may place a cushion between your buttocks and your heels if this is more comfortable. Use Reverse Breathing (1) to pull up your perineum, bring your waist back, open your chest and "sit tall".

44 Kneel tall

In this dynamic version of Vajrasana, left, the flow of breath assists the lift of the diaphragm in a rhythmical stretch up and down.

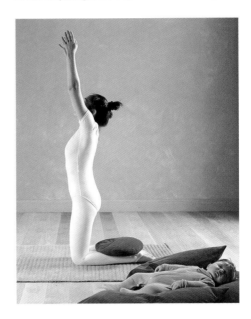

◁ Bring your hands together in front of you. As you breathe in, raise your buttocks, keeping your spine vertical and tailbone tucked under, and lift your arms above your head. Breathe out as you sit back. Breathe in and rise again and, if you can, hold for a few breaths before sitting back.

45 Chest expansion

This exercise is both a stretch and a forward bend. The challenge is to find the position in which your arms can stretch the most while your chest can open the widest. Make sure your neck remains relaxed throughout.

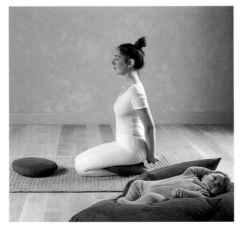

△ **1** Clasp your hands behind your back, sitting tall. Bring your arms up behind you, keeping them as straight as possible and squeezing your shoulder blades together.

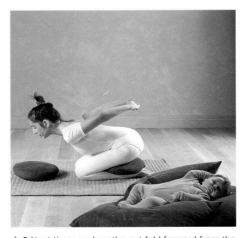

△ **2** Next time you breathe out fold forward from the hips, keeping your arms raised. Breathe in, sitting tall. On the out-breath, fold forward from the hips and lift your clasped hands, opening your chest as wide as possible. Keep expanding forward, breathing as deeply as possible.

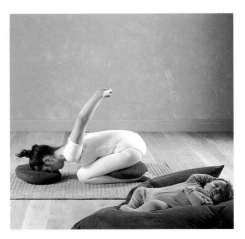

△ **3** Aim to place your head on the floor (or cushion) in front of you, while still sitting on your heels. Breathe deeply and work to bring your arms higher with each breath out. Release your hands and come up on an in-breath, sitting quietly in Vajrasana and observing the effects of the last exercise.

46 Kneeling twist

Twisting in Vajrasana is slightly more difficult than the sitting twists on a chair presented earlier (17–19). Make sure you can kneel comfortably, with a straight spine, before you practise this kneeling twist. It allows further rotation and therefore is stimulating and enjoyable, even more so when you add a circling movement of the shoulder.

▷ **1** Place the back of one hand against the outside of the opposite knee and the other hand on the floor behind you. These are your levers. Sit up very straight as you breathe in and turn as you breathe out. Improve your twist with successive breaths out. Keep your neck relaxed and only turn your head to the extent that your spine twists. Eventually, you find yourself looking backwards without strain.

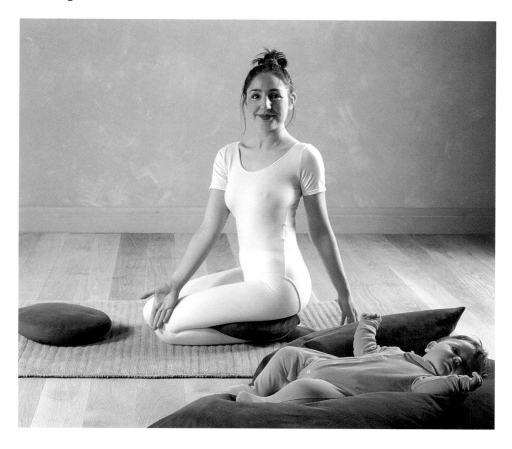

◁ **2** When you are ready, bend your back elbow and put your fingertips on your shoulder. Circle your elbow, loosening your shoulder and upper back. Repeat on the other side.

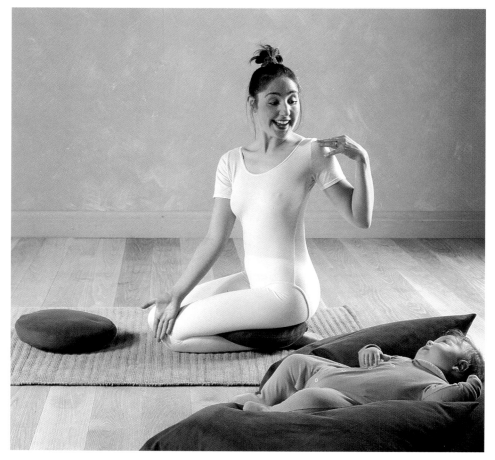

"Look at today for it is life.

The very life of life."

Kneeling roll

This sequence offers an expanded version of the Cat Pose (25). It is a stepping stone between the full "kneeling sun salute" (24–26) which keeps you grounded in your practice, and the classic sun salute of all yoga schools. We are giving a great deal of attention to this sequence because if it is not done correctly you may weaken your lumbar area when you move on to the full sun salute. Make sure you use your breath fully in time with the rhythm of this exercise, which is known as the "kneeling wheel".

47 Rhythmic kneeling sequence

Repeat this rhythmic, rolling movement several times to loosen and relax your whole spine. The sequence is based on the Cat Pose (25), kneeling on all fours. Check that your knees are directly under your hips, hip-width apart, and that your hands are under your shoulder joints.

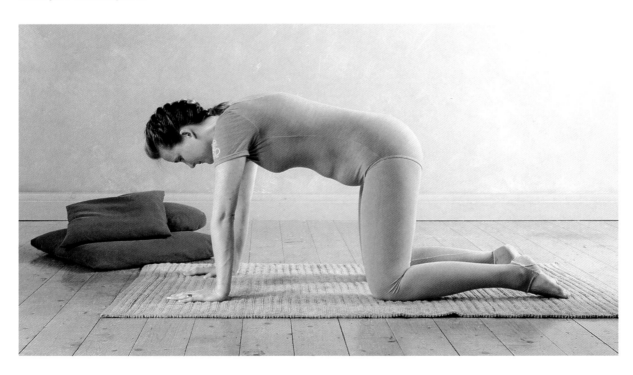

◁ **1** Begin with your back flat, with your neck and spine in a straight line. If you wish, practise the Cat Pose (25) first, stretching and arching your spine alternately on the in- and out-breath.

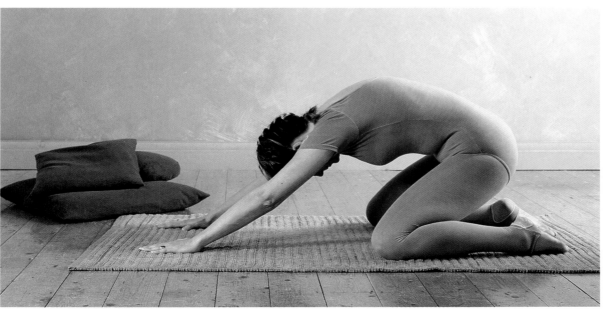

◁ **2** Lean back as you breathe out, opening up the lower back. Keep your arms fully extended (your hands have not moved at all) and lower your head as you stretch back. Ideally, your head comes to touch the floor while you remain seated on your heels.

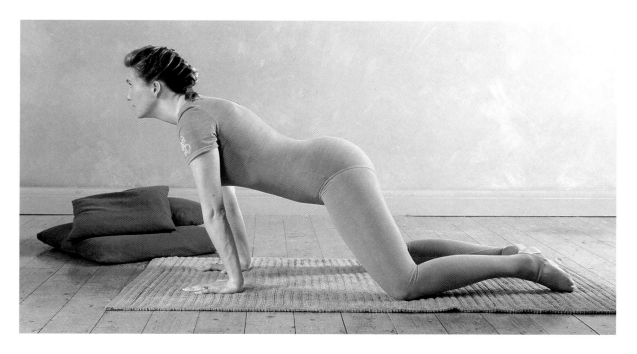

◁ **3** Inhale, extending forward on your knees and bent arms until you have to straighten your arms and raise your head to come up, moving your weight on your hands and lifting your shoulders.

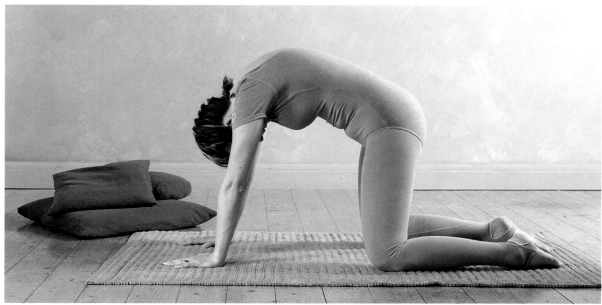

◁ **4** As soon as you reach the limit of both your in-breath and your stretch, start rolling your shoulders to extend backwards with your arms straight on a long out-breath.

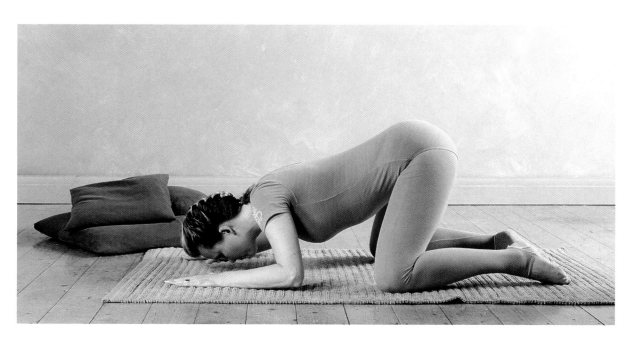

◁ **5** At the end of your out-breath, you are ready to bring your elbows to the floor again and start stretching forward on a new in-breath, extending your back fully again, as above. Keep your head relaxed. Enjoy the "wheel" movement with the flow of the breath in and out. Then relax.

From kneeling to sitting

From kneeling in Vajrasana (43), on your heels (or on a cushion placed on your heels) you can now move on to Virasana, a pose in which you sit between your heels (or on a cushion between your heels). This pose tones your abdominal muscles further and allows you to make Reverse Breathing (1) even more effective. You can use it as a base to stretch backwards and up. Virasana makes sitting straight in Dandasana easier as well as preparing you for the forward bends of classic yoga with a fully extended back.

48 Virasana

For this classical yoga kneeling pose you sit between your feet. If you find this pose difficult, place rolled cushions between your thighs and sit on these – it will get easier with practice.

▷ From a kneeling position, adjust yourself to make a comfortable descent towards a cushion or the floor, supporting yourself with your hands as you lower your buttocks between your feet. Make sure you can sit straight. Practise Reverse Breathing (1) in this position.

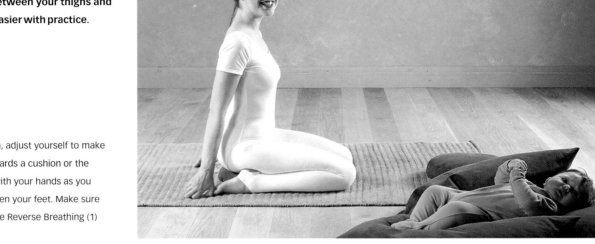

49 Back arch

Virasana allows you a full expansion of the chest and a stretch of the spine by moving your hands back in an easy back arch.

50 Push away

An upward stretch in Virasana knits your right abdominal muscles back together after pregnancy. If these muscles have split, practise this pose frequently for repair.

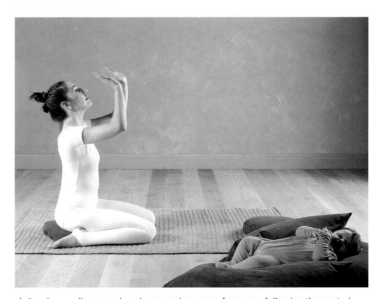

△ Breathe in and, as you breathe out, take your hands back with the fingers pointing forwards. Lower your weight on to your palms and breathe in deeply to open the chest and arch the spine. Take several deep breaths in this pose. Come out of it as you went in, crawling your fingers back towards your buttocks.

△ Bend your elbows and push your palms away from you, following the seated sequence described in detail in the Sun Wheel Stretch (16). This exercise is very effective to tone your right abdominal muscles. Exhale slowly on the way up, breathing in before you start pushing again from below.

51 Dandasana

This is a classical yoga sitting position. The word means "pose of a stick". You can use it to stretch your spine and legs before you relax after completing a sequence of kneeling poses. Put on some more clothes, so that you don't get cold, and place a beanbag, or a big pile of cushions, in position.

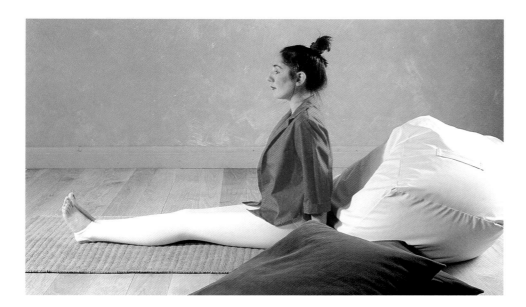

◁ **1** Sit close to the beanbag. Stretch your legs out, with your feet flexed. Place your hands near your buttocks and use them to push your spine upright and at a right angle to your straight legs. Use Reverse Breathing (1) to help you lengthen your lower back. Feel how you are sitting up taller and taller as you breathe. Your leg muscles are also toning as you lift yourself more from your buttock bones on the floor.

▷**2** Raise your arms on an in breath and push away with your palms as you exhale, keeping your head relaxed. Bend your arms again as you inhale and push them further up as you exhale. This is a graceful but very demanding rhythmical stretch in which nearly every muscle in your body gets involved! If you find sitting on the floor too difficult for now, sit on a cushion or on the edge of a beanbag.

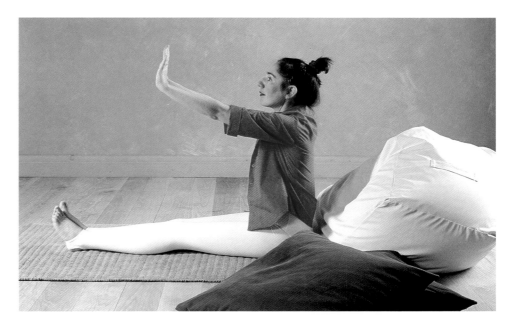

▽ **3** When you feel really stretched lie back on the beanbag and totally let go... perhaps alone, perhaps with company.

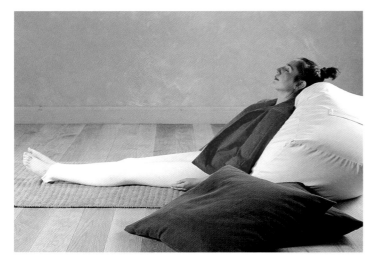

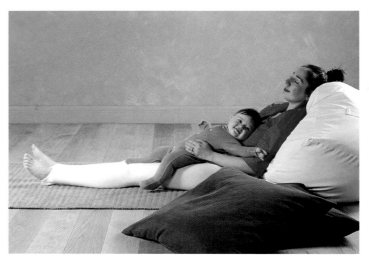

Making yoga part of your life

The breathing, movements and relaxation that make up your yoga practice will extend naturally into your everyday life. Take a few moments at frequent intervals to check the pattern of your breathing, the sense of "energy flow" in your movements and the state of relaxed contentment in your heart and mind. Make yoga a part of your life with a few appropriate exercises, wherever you happen to be.

At this stage your life is becoming more outward-looking, as you begin to resume your normal interests outside the home and you may be preparing to go back to work. You need flexible daily routines that suit your baby, your family and yourself.

Caring for yourself is still important. Maintain a special place in your own home where you can turn inward in deep relaxation to address concerns and feelings that are very personal. Your "yoga corner" can become the projection of your inner space, as you and your baby transform week by week.

When you nurture yourself during deep relaxation, you also strengthen the bond with your baby and dissolve stress around you. Yoga practice can become the tool for your transformation into a well-adapted mother. Whether you are at home or at work, you can refresh yourself daily.

52 Carrying

When you are sitting on a chair with your baby on your lap you can practise "pelvic rolls" to ease out your lower back and gain flexibility and awareness in this area. Use them to help you get up from the chair, and practise the same movements in reverse every time you sit down. They can also be used to get in and out of cars.

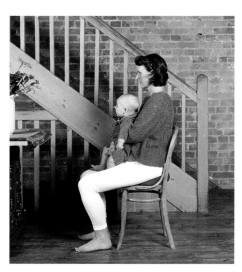

◁ **1** Arch your lower back, then tuck your tailbone under. Repeat this in a rolling action.

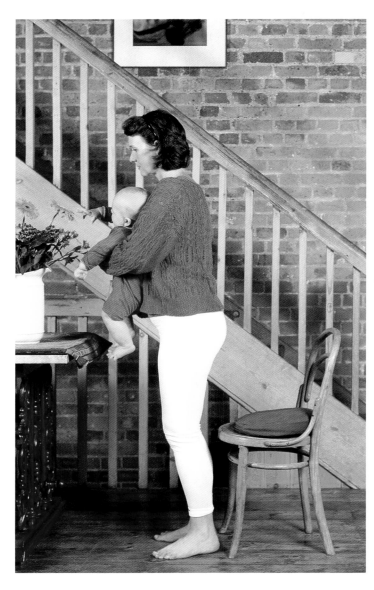

◁ **2** When you stand up while carrying your baby, tuck your tailbone under and bend your knees while keeping your back straight.

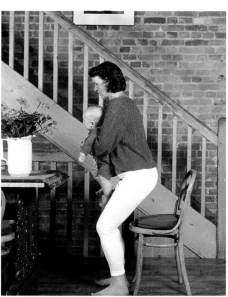

▷ **3** Let your thighs carry your weight, while your arms and upper back carry your baby.

53 Easy lifting

Use this technique for heavy shopping, but remember that babies in seats also constitute heavy loads, and they get heavier as they grow. So you will feel much more comfortable if you apply the principles of yoga from the start.

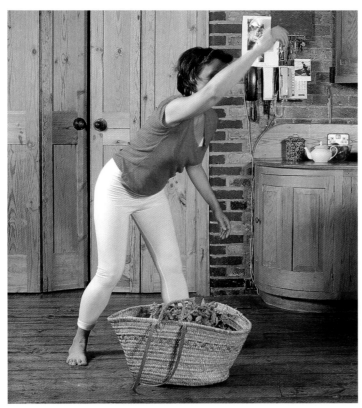

△ **1** To loosen up, bend your knees then straighten your legs as you stretch one arm, or both arms. Bend again as you release your arm or arms, and continue swinging in a rhythm; inhale as you stretch, exhale as you release.

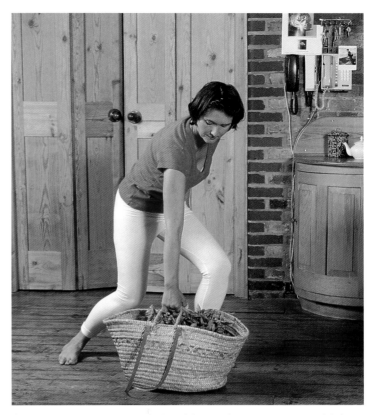

△ **2** Pick up your load at the beginning of the upswing movement, as you inhale. Before lifting, your legs are bent and your arm is relaxed.

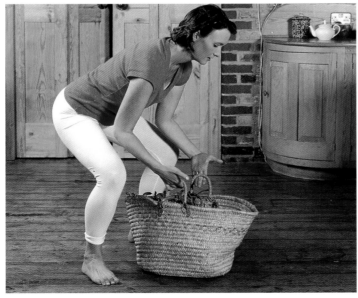

△ **3** If you are lifting a heavy load, always use both hands. Again, make sure that you are on the upswing, with your legs bent and your arms relaxed, beginning your inhalation. Feel that your abdominal muscles are involved, but do not strain.

▷ **4** Lift as you inhale, keeping your knees bent and your back straight. You may find this makes greater use of your arm muscles, but your back is protected. Put a heavy load down in the same way, but in reverse order, breathing out as you let go of it. Relax your lower back and abdomen as you exhale (all the way down).

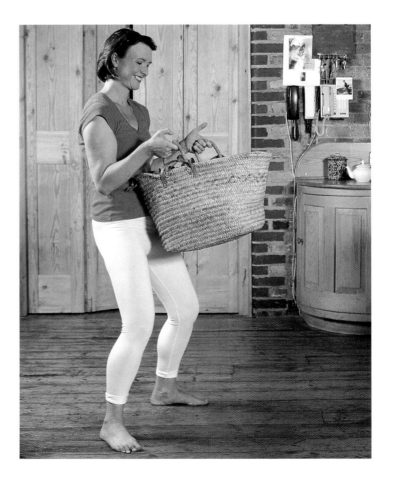

Yoga up and down stairs

gentle progression

Unless you live in a bungalow, you will find yourself going upstairs and downstairs many times a day with your baby. You may also have to carry piles of linen and clothes, and Moses basket, carry cot or baby seat. This sequence will help you to protect your back and also to stretch your spine as you go up and down. Make the stairs a prop to regain or gain fitness each day, with yoga.

54 Stairs

Going up and down the stairs, bending and extending your legs while keeping your back straight can make a striking difference to your energy level at the end of the day.

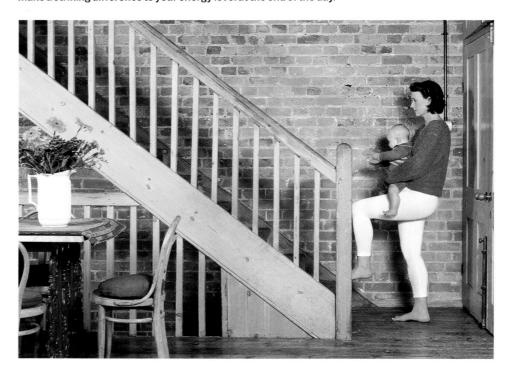

▷ **1** Going up, lift your bent knee really high and stretch up before you take your weight on your top foot. With practice, you can learn to inhale as you bend and exhale as you stretch.

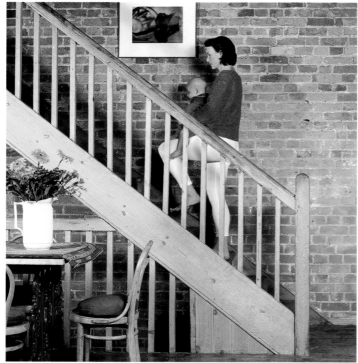

△ **2** Practise shifting your weight from your stretched back leg to your front bent leg, extending your leg muscles fully as you go upstairs. Keep your back straight.

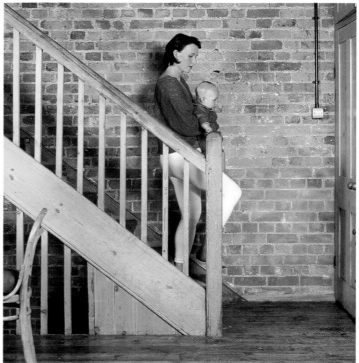

△ **3** Going down, bend your knees deeply, keeping your back straight all the time. Inhale as you lift your knee, before lowering your leg down to the next step on the out-breath.

55 Swing on the bannister

These stretches expand the movements that you make while going upstairs and downstairs. Practise them while leaning on a bannister or a table. They will strengthen your lower back and legs to walk upstairs and downstairs without strain.

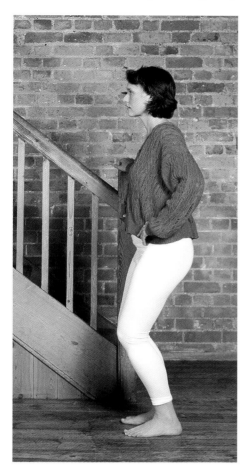

◁ **1** Starting in Tadasana (28), bend your knees, keeping your back as straight as possible. Have your hands on your hips or hold on to the bannister with one hand. Go down on an out-breath, extend back up on an in-breath.

▷ **2** From the same starting point, swing your left bent knee as high as you can on an in-breath. Keep your standing leg slightly flexed. Let your leg go down to the floor softly as you exhale and push with your foot on an in-breath to swing your bent leg up again. Repeat a few times then change legs.

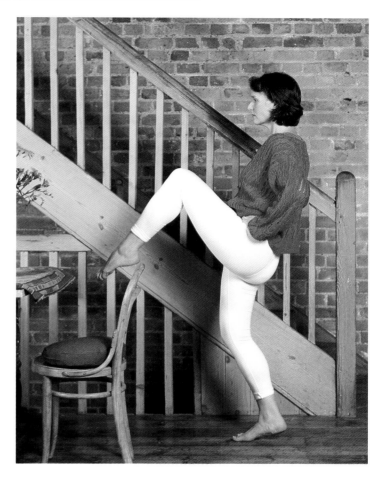

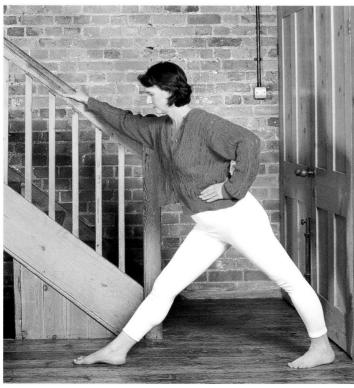

△ **3** Stand on the side of the bannister with your legs extended in a wide step, turning your back foot slightly outward. Stretch your arm on the side of your front leg, using the bannister, on an in-breath.

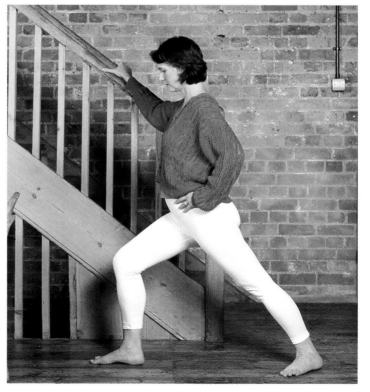

△ **4** On the out-breath, bend your knee and allow your lower back to stretch. This is an easy static version of the Walking Warrior (42). Change sides. Use any convenient support if you do not have a bannister.

Family yoga

When your yoga becomes an integral part of how you move, breathe, think and feel, then every space can be a yoga space for you. You are now ready to include others in your practice from time to time.

It can be great fun to practise together as a family and keeps siblings and the father involved with you and the new baby. It is best to keep the sessions short and choose simple exercises that children find fun to do. There should be no attempt to achieve a "perfect" pose, even if there is actually such a thing. The breadth and depth of awareness and steadiness that can be achieved in yoga seem to be unlimited. For occasional sessions with mixed ages and mixed abilities, focus on being relaxed, moving from one pose to the next as the energy flows. Lead them by your example, avoid explanation and don't hold any position. Above all, hand out heaps of praise!

" Little one, I embrace your presence in my life, my togetherness with you. When were you not a part of my life and my heart?"

There are times when family practice seems to be the only alternative to abandoning your practice altogether, or carrying on through gritted teeth, trying strenuously to ignore any interruptions. This attitude will spoil your yoga practice, as well as unsettling your nervous system. So make a virtue of necessity, take a deep breath and invite the family to join in. Choose a pose that is suitable for them and also totally familiar to you. Show them how to do it by demonstrating it in a smiling and relaxed manner. Do it with them a few times. Then move on to another pose. When they get bored you can go back to your own yoga practice, still in a serene and happy mood.

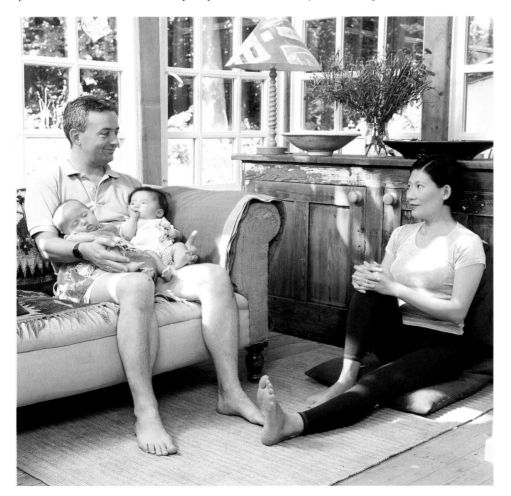

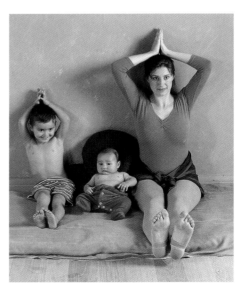

△ **The example of your breathing helps your children to breathe more deeply.**

◁ **While you may feel that your partner's life is relatively unchanged while yours is so different now, doing yoga with him or next to him can be quality time.**

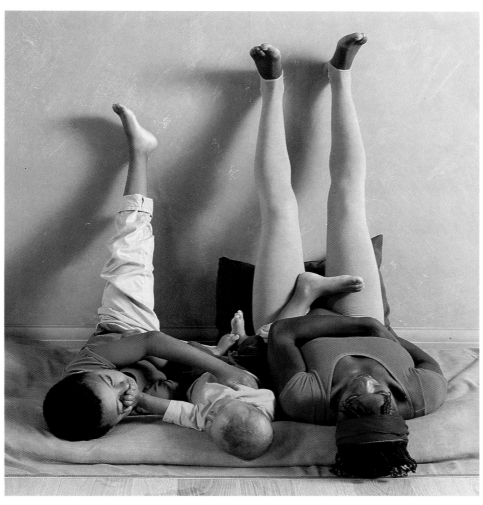

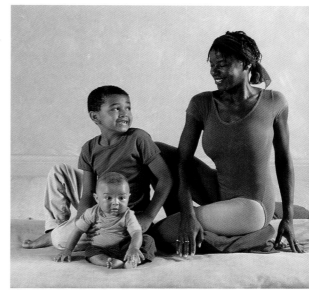

△ Children like the challenge of simple yoga positions. Help them copy your movements as accurately as possible without strain.

◁ Time to rest with your Legs up the Wall (5). Every moment can also be playtime.

▽ Older children can benefit greatly from joining in and trying some of the new mother's stretches!

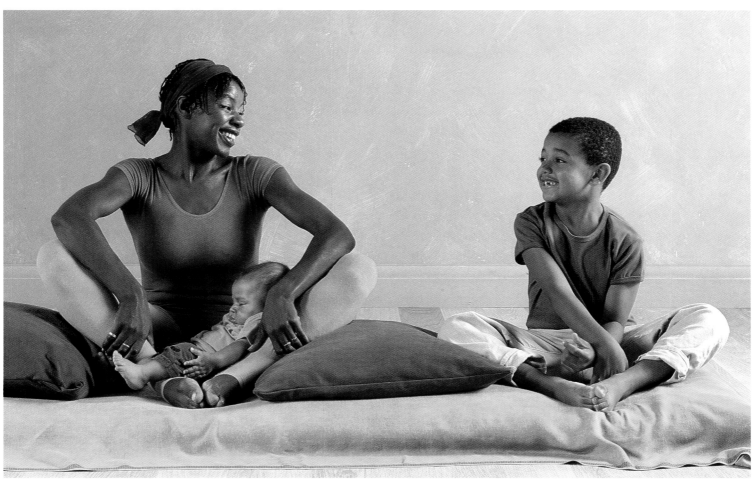

Yoga with friends

It makes an interesting change to practise yoga with friends, at your home or theirs. It is always fun for mothers and babies to get together. Most babies are fascinated with other babies, so it will make your own life much easier in the future if you introduce your baby to a number of different (and friendly) people and places as early in life as possible. Your baby will build up trust

and confidence through experiencing a variety of different people and faces from the earliest days.

Women who first meet during their pregnancies can become friends for life. They enjoy the fun times together and give each other mutual support through any hard and lonely times. They may also start going to yoga classes together.

There are many exercises you can do with a partner. Be inventive, yet careful. It can be very easy for the "helper" to strain the lower back. As a general rule, let the floor support the weight, rather than either partner. Friends who do yoga together will benefit from the symmetry of postures. Make sure you communicate well so that you both feel equally stretched.

56 Leg and arm stretches

This is a good routine to enjoy with a partner. Sit facing each other on a mat, a little more than a leg's length apart. Through mutual pushing and pulling of arms and then legs in symmetrical dynamic postures, you both energize and have good fun.

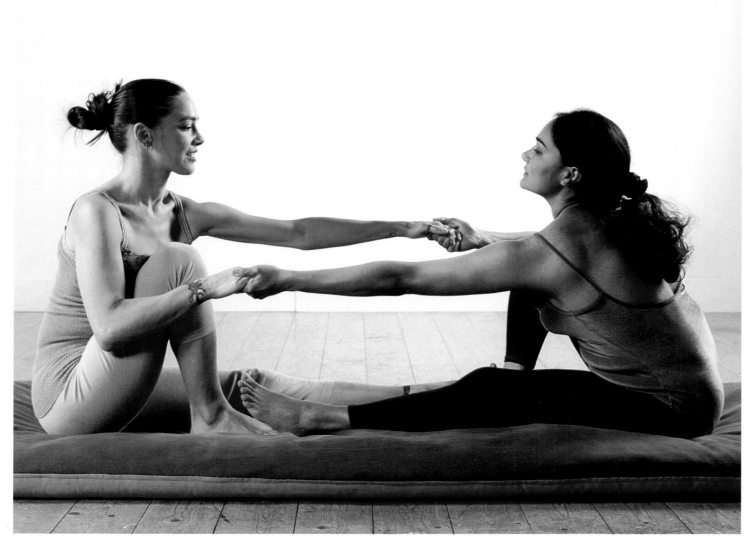

△ **1** Each of you bends the right knee and the right elbow, as you hold hands. Sit up straight, adjusting the distance between you until you are both in a firm sitting position with your arms at shoulder level. Now twist your upper bodies by bending/extending your arms alternately in an easy rhythm. Change legs. Breathe in the rhythm.

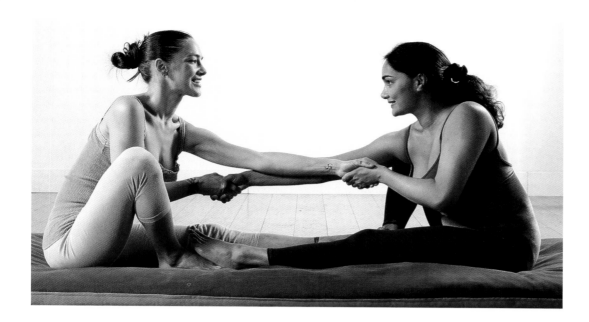

◁ **2** Change your hand hold, so that you are reaching to clasp your partner's opposite hand.

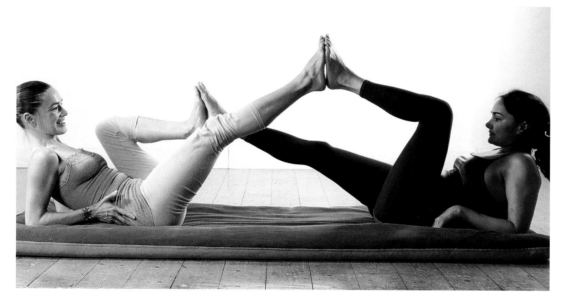

◁ **3** Now work your legs. Lean back on to your forearms and bring the soles of your feet against those of your partner. Keeping contact, "cycle" with your legs – forwards a few times, then backwards.

▽**4** Finish by sitting back to back, using the pressure of your partner's back against your own to achieve a beautiful Dandasana pose (51). Keep your feet flexed and hold the position, breathing deeply and in unison. This breathing together is bonding, and your babies will feel very comfortable sharing the atmosphere that you are radiating.

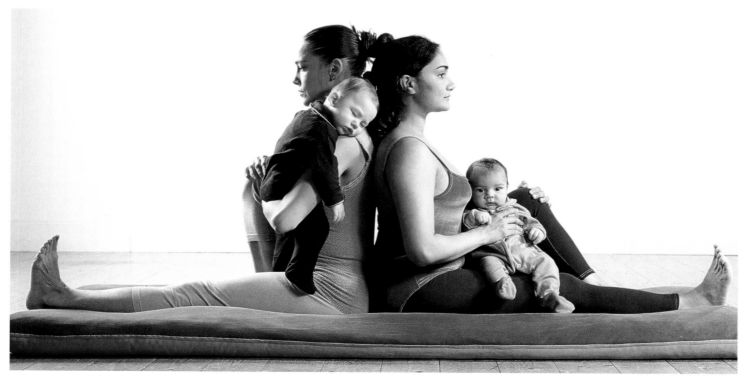

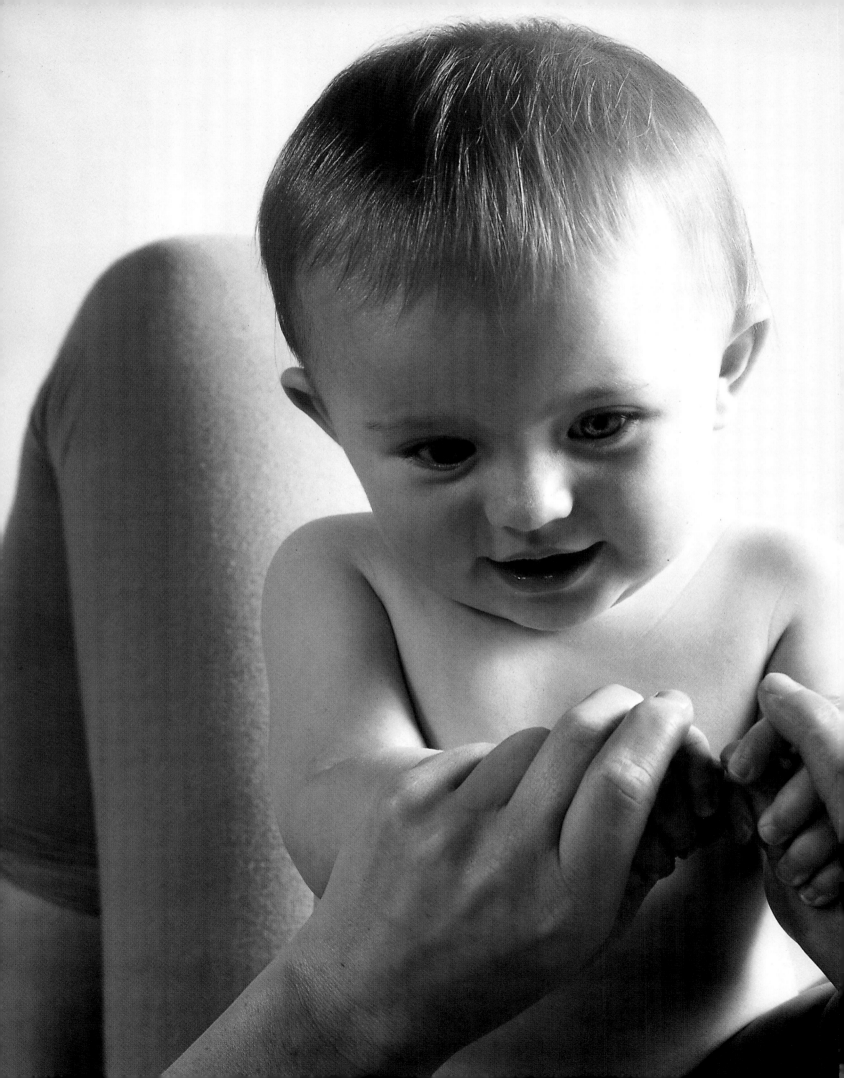

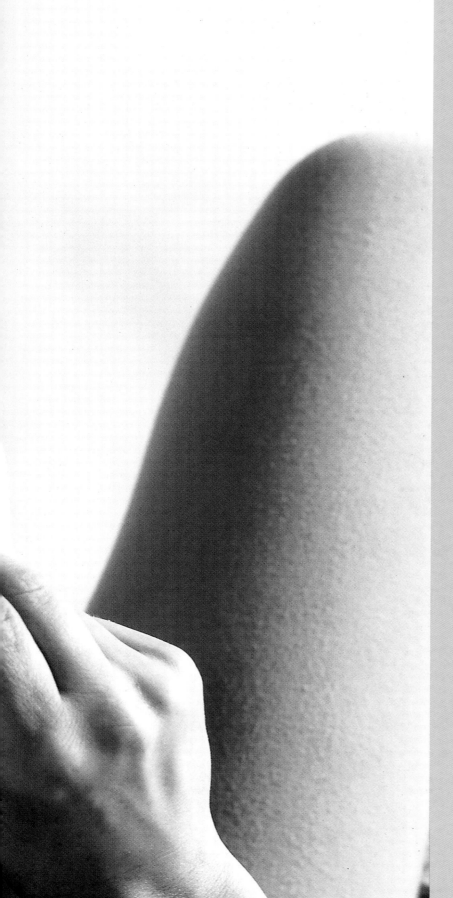

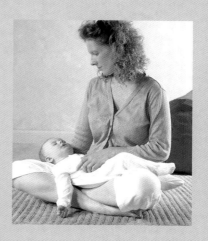

gaining
strength

The feel-good factor of gentle yoga is
expanded by the regular practice of
movements and postures that increase new
mothers' energy and enjoyment of life day
by day. This is the time to replenish or
renew your vitality, gaining stamina while
remaining centred in mindfulness. Watch
your baby copying you!

Three to six months after birth

This section continues to develop a solid foundation for long-term good posture, pelvic strength and suppleness after your pregnancy and birth. Now is the time for you to influence the state of your hips and your lower back over many years to come. With yoga, you can continue benefitting from the flexibility that the hormones of pregnancy have given you, without over-stretching too soon. The aims are to strengthen and elongate the spinal muscles in your re-aligned body.

The asanas in this section cater both for those experienced in yoga and for those new to it. You are progressively introduced to classical poses in which the hips are aligned in stretches, twists and bends with the legs open in a wide step forward. While these poses are easy if you have done yoga, you may find breathing deeply in them a new challenge. If you are new to yoga, then getting correctly into the poses as shown here will be your first step.

Once again, this time-scheme is only a general guide. You may feel more comfortable sticking with the earlier routines for a while longer. You may also prefer to take one pose at a time from this section and practise it together with earlier, already familiar poses. It is always best to proceed at your own pace, consolidating your gains and enjoying your progress.

"You are the bows from which

your children as living arrows

are sent forth."

The Prophet

57 "Easy" Warrior

This pose gives you back strong, masculine energy which you may welcome to balance the yielding and softening needed to welcome your newborn. It helps you to feel "back in your body" and makes you firm, vigorous and strong with breathing in the abdomen, solar plexus and heart combined. The Walking Warrior (42) can still be useful when your baby is awake and wanting your company. Use this standing pose to improve the walking version.

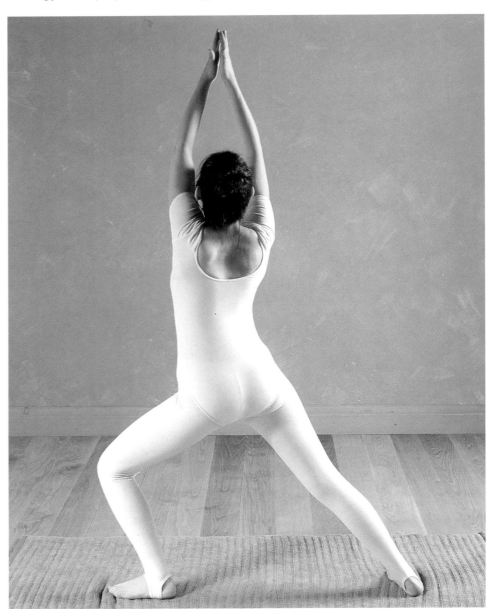

△ Stand with your legs apart and turn one foot to the side as for the "Easy" Triangle Pose (Trikonasana) (36), keeping your trunk facing to the front. Breathing in deeply, bring your arms overhead with palms together in a strong, vigorous lift of the upper body. Breathing naturally, improve your position. Open your chest and bring your shoulder blades closer together. Look straight ahead, keeping your chin level and your ears in line with your shoulders. Straighten your arms. When you are ready, breathe out and bend your front knee, keeping your spine erect and weight centred. Breathe in the pose for a moment, then breathe in to straighten your knee and out to lower your arms. If you are experienced in yoga, turn your trunk forward in a classic Warrior Pose.

58 Triangle forward bend (Parsvottanasana)

This pose combines a stretch, a twist and a bend. The more slowly you extend and the more fully you breathe, with your awareness on the base of the spine, the greater appreciation you will get of the calm strength you gain from this pose.

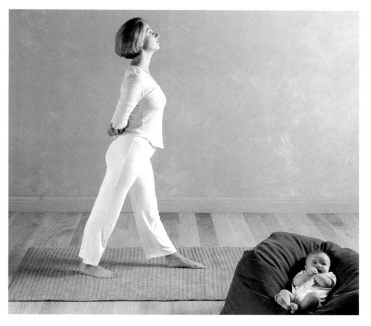

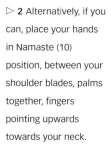 **1** Start in Tadasana (28). Take a comfortable step forward and turn your back foot out, keeping your weight on the back heel. Clasp both elbows behind your back.

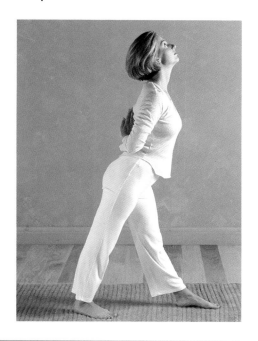

▷ **2** Alternatively, if you can, place your hands in Namaste (10) position, between your shoulder blades, palms together, fingers pointing upwards towards your neck.

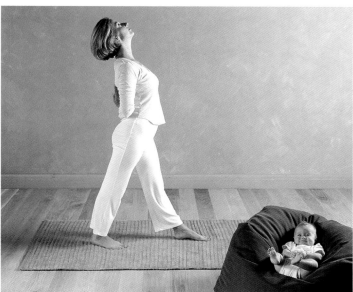

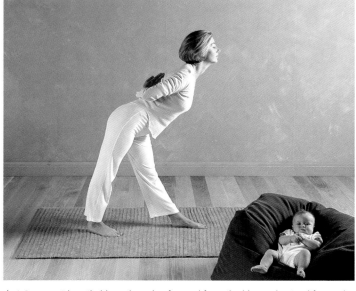

△ **3** Stretch up and back, all the way from your front foot to the top of your head, breathing in slowly and keeping your weight on your back heel. Take a few deep breaths while stretching.

△ **4** On an out-breath, hinge the spine forward from the hips and extend forward slowly, taking a few deep breaths and lifting your breastbone. When you cannot extend any further, drop your head.

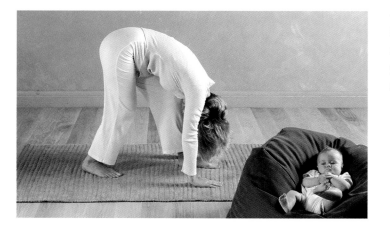

◁ **5** If you are experienced in yoga, allow your forehead to rest on your front knee, keeping your weight on the back heel. If this is too difficult, loosen your arms and bring your hands forward, palms on the floor, flexing the knees if needed, to keep your back extended in the forward bend. From either position, come back up slowly, taking a few deep breaths.

Elongating the spine

As you go through successive stages of feeling aligned and stronger after giving birth, it is a pleasure to recover, or perhaps discover, the joy of stretching your spine. These deceptively simple adapted yoga poses make use of a support – a chair here – to help you enjoy the benefits of a fully stretched back. Feel the downward pull of gravity and the uplift in your lower back.

59 Leg-up sequence

This is harder than it looks! Find a support for your leg at a height that suits your physique and level of fitness – from low to high chair, to table top.

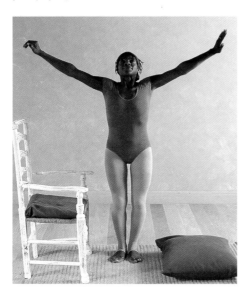

◁ **1** To begin, stand in Tadasana (28) and circle your straight arms in wide backward sweeps, lifting in the waist, breathing freely.

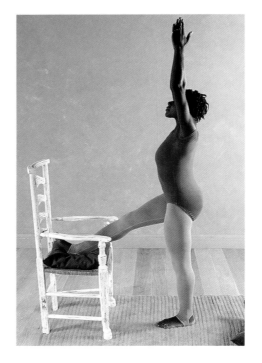

◁ **2** When you feel loosened up and stretched, place one leg on the chair with the knee straight and the foot flexed. Regain a balanced and upright posture and bring your palms to face each other overhead. Stretch up more on each breath out, squeezing in at the waist. Hold the position for three to five breaths. Relax your leg. Then change legs and repeat.

60 Open twist

A standing version of the sitting twist, this pose uses movement to prepare you for the classic Standing Twist (66).

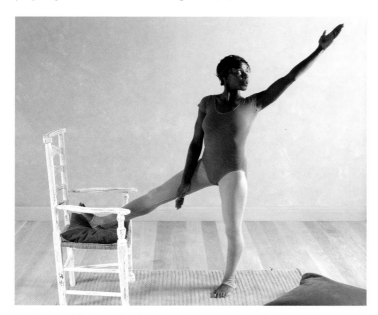

△ With your right leg on the chair, place the corresponding hand on the inner side of your thigh as a lever and twist, circling your straight arm. While opening the chest wide, this pose allows a stretch from the standing leg to the extended hand.

61 Closed twist (2)

In this twisting stretch, the pressure of the hand on the outer side of the raised leg allows a rotation of the hips.

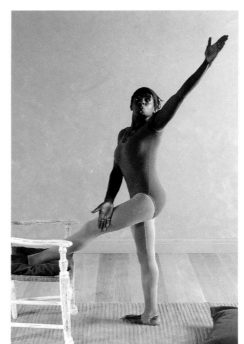

◁ When you twist to the left this time, your leg is on the chair and the back of your right hand is the lever against the outside of your left thigh. Circle your left arm several times in wide upward and backward sweeps, lifting at the waist. Twist both sides equally.

62 Forward bend (2)

The raised leg helps you find more extension in the back as you bend forward, breathing as deeply in your lower abdomen as possible. Open the backs of the knees and enjoy aligning your hips for further stretch.

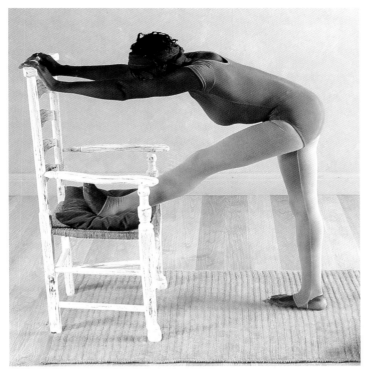

△ **1** Rest one straight leg on the chair with the foot flexed. Pull your spine up tall and raise both arms slowly overhead, palms facing each other. Stretch with the breath, then, on an out-breath, hinge forward from the hips with a straight and stretched spine. Hold on to the back of the chair and breathe freely.

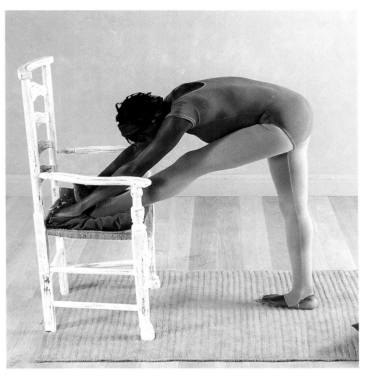

△ **2** Alternatively, hold your foot. Keep your legs straight and make sure that your neck and head remain relaxed as you extend in the forward bend. Keep the hip of the raised leg pulled back.

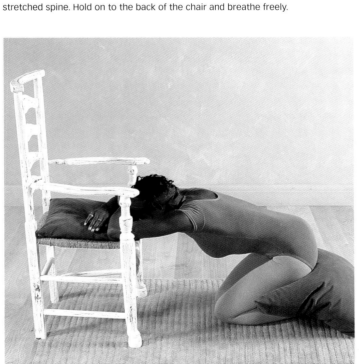

△ **3** To rest after these stretches, kneel down in front of the chair, with a cushion between your heels and your buttocks if you wish, and rest your folded arms on the chair seat. Breathe deeply into your back to relax.

63 Upper back strengthener

This exercise continues toning your central, vertical abdominal muscles as well as strengthening the upper back.

▷ Sit in an upright chair and raise your baby high above your head as you inhale. Lower the baby slowly into your lap as you exhale, remembering to use your abdominal muscles as you breathe. Repeat whenever you have a spare moment.

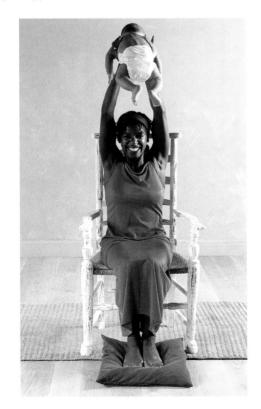

More kitchen yoga

Mothers spend a great deal of time in the kitchen, which often becomes the focus of the home with babies and small children around. However small your kitchen or living area may be, you are likely to have a sink, counter or table which will become an invaluable prop for your yoga practice. These exercises can be done at odd moments when you feel the need for a good stretch.

64 Table top spine

This and the following two stretches involve using a table or counter that is the right height for your legs and current flexibility. For this stretch, it is better for the surface to be too high than too low. It takes considerable awareness to get your spine in a straight line. Start by standing tall in Tadasana (28).

▷ **1** Put your hands on the table, bend at the hips and walk backwards as far as you can, until your spine is stretching horizontally. Avoid sagging in the middle, dropping your head or hunching your shoulders. Ask someone else to tell you where you are not as straight as you could be, and to put a hand on the spot so that you know where to adjust.

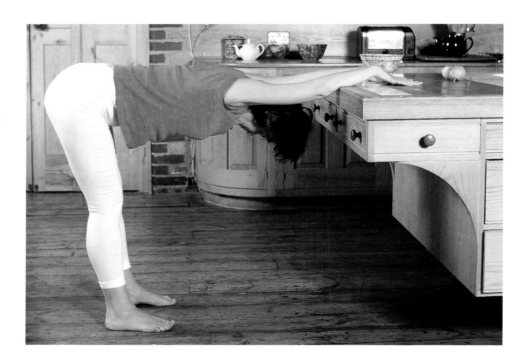

▷ **2** To get more stretch, bend your knees and pull the base of the spine further away from your shoulders. Sway your hips right and left, or even circle them with your knees bent to give your lower back a complete stretch.

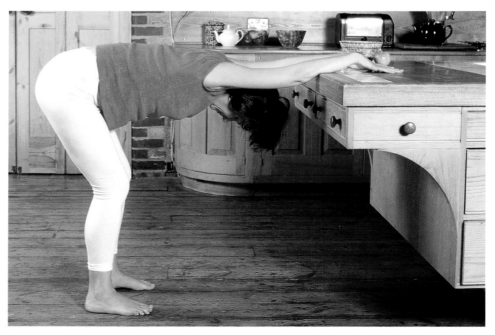

"Ever serenely balanced, I am neither free nor bound." *Song of the Soul*

65 Leg lift

As you are getting stronger, you can use an extended leg, with a support under the foot, to stretch, bend and twist in a standing posture. This sequence looks deceptively easy (it is an intensive toner of your inner thighs and buttocks). See also 22, 75, 76, 77.

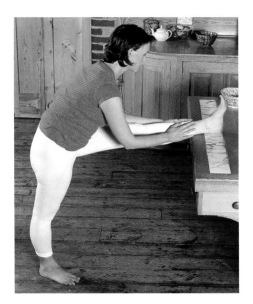

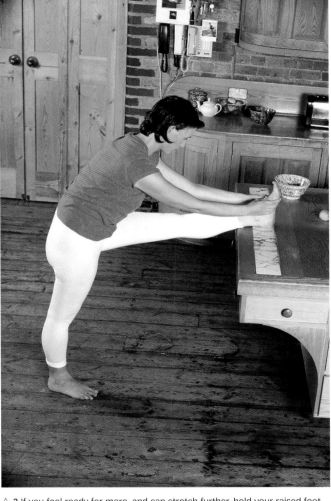

◁ **1** If you feel energetic, place one leg on a chair, counter or table. It is better to have it too low than too high for this exercise. Have both legs straight. Your standing leg should be right under your hip. Flex the foot of the raised leg.

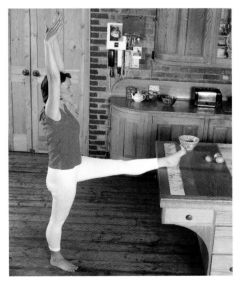

◁ **2** On an in-breath, raise both arms straight above your head. Exhale and stretch more. Take a few deep breaths in this position before lowering your arms on an out-breath. After releasing your arms, bend forward from the hips, sliding your hands down your leg, on an out-breath. Slide a little further in the next out-breath, extending your lower back. Keep your head relaxed.

△ **3** If you feel ready for more, and can stretch further, hold your raised foot with both hands, keeping your arms and head as relaxed as possible. Inhale and bend forward loosely on the exhale. Come up and rest your legs or move on to the leg twist. Change leg.

66 Standing twist

This is a standing version of the twists shown before, in both Sitting (17) and Kneeling (46) positions. A standing twist adds a further stretch in the leg and buttock muscles to the rotation of the spine from the base.

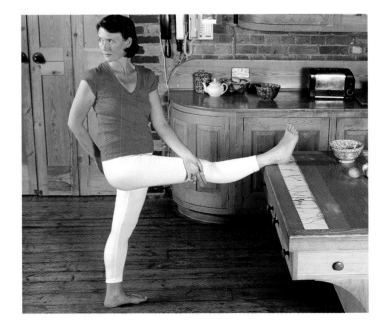

◁ With your right leg on the table, place the back of your left hand against the outside of your right thigh and the back of the right hand behind your waist. These are your two levers. Breathe in. Pull the spine up, opening and lifting the chest as you rotate slowly on the out-breath. Breathe in again and twist further to the right. Repeat to the left.

Kneeling balance

As you progress in your yoga practice, make up your own routine, integrating new positions in the first basic sequences. This kneeling balance allows you to experience the full stretch which you will gain later from classic standing balances, while still remaining grounded on one hand and one knee. Balances will help you regain lightness and agility after pregnancy.

67 Cat balance

This is a wonderful stretch, which you can do after completing the Rhythmic Kneeling Sequence (47). Begin in the Cat Pose (25), kneeling on all fours with your knees directly under your hips and your hands under your shoulders.

▷ **1** With your neck and spine aligned, raise one arm and the opposite leg, making a straight line from hand to foot. Hold the position, breathing deeply, then repeat on the other side.

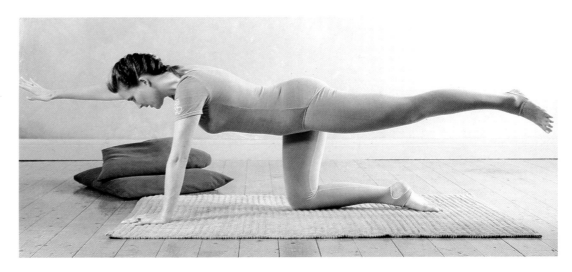

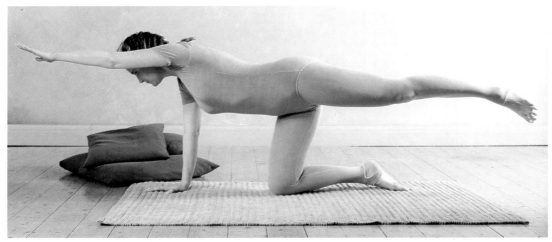

◁ **2** Now raise the arm and leg on the same side and stretch out straight. Hold, breathing deeply. Feel a stretch down from the hip to the foot and a stretch up from the waist to the hand, creating further space for breathing into. Repeat on the other side.

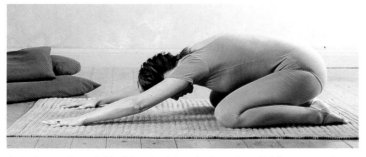

△ **3** When you have finished, lean back into the Swan Pose (24) for a moment.

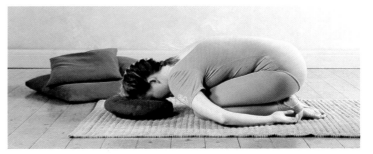

△ **4** Or, bringing your arms beside your body, relax in what is known as the Child Pose, breathing deeply. You may like to place a cushion under your forehead.

Shoulder stretch

The feeding of your baby is well established by now, whether you are still breastfeeding or bottle-feeding at this stage. It is time to stretch anew your arms, shoulders and neck, stimulating the flow of energy in your heart and throat Chakras. The following exercises tone the muscles that support your breasts. They stimulate the production of milk if you are breastfeeding.

68 Routine for shoulders and neck

You have already practised some of these movements separately. Do them as a sequence whenever your shoulders and neck feel tight, tense or sore. Start by loosening your shoulders and neck, sitting in Vajrasana (43): between your heels, with your big toes touching each other. If you need to, put a cushion between your heels and your buttocks.

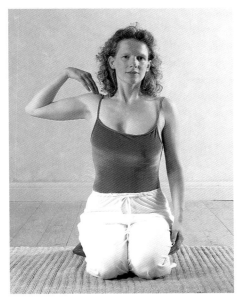

◁ **1** Place the fingertips of one hand on your shoulder and circle your elbow several times in each direction.

▷ **2** Repeat with the other arm, then circle both elbows together. Keep your spine stretched tall and your chest open throughout.

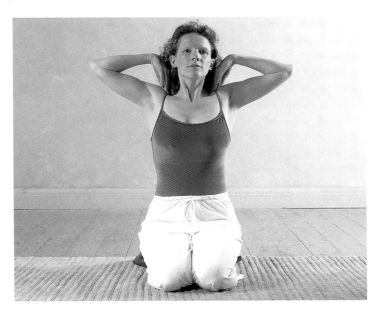

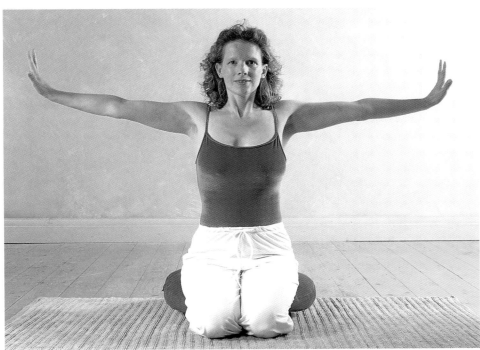

△ **3** Now push your palms out in a kneeling version of the "Sun Wheel" Stretch (16), straightening your arms as you push away, breathing out, and bending your elbows as you bring them in, breathing in.

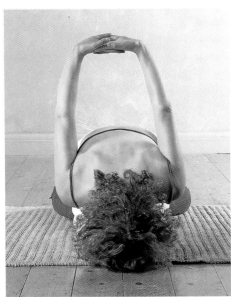

△ **4** Clasp your hands behind you for the Chest Expansion (45), and bring your head to the floor in front of you. Hold the position for several deep breaths, then release your hands and bring your arms beside you in the Child Pose (opposite).

Sitting poses

After giving birth, some women find that they are less flexible in the hip joints, while others feel they have gained flexibility.

Whatever is the case for you, sitting poses allow you to elongate and strengthen your spine in a variety of ways. As you stretch, bend

and twist with your legs in different positions, your "sit-bones" are your anchor on the floor and the root of your spinal stretch.

69 Seated forward bend (Paschimottanasana)

Start by sitting tall, with your legs straight in front of you in Dandasana (51), extending from your seat to your crown with your shoulders and head relaxed. Always think of extending with an in-breath before you bend on an out-breath. If you cannot bend forward without your knees coming up or your abdomen getting squashed, use a belt or a tie round your feet.

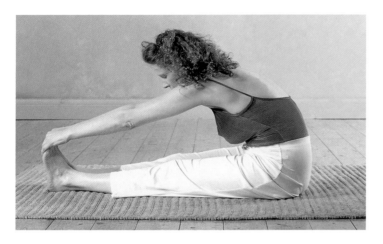

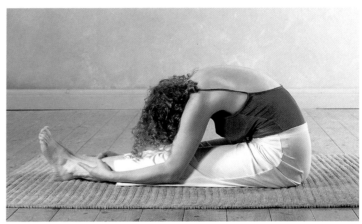

△ **1** Inhale to stretch up your spine. As you exhale, lengthen forward from the hips to reach your toes, or whichever part of your leg you can reach without strain. Keep extending the back of your knees.

△ **2** If this is comfortable, relax by bending your elbows and placing your forearms on the floor alongside your shins. Feel your hips go down on the floor as you extend your spine further with each exhalation.

70 Foot to the side forward bend (Trianga Mukhaikapada Paschimottasana) (TMP)

This is an asymmetric forward bend, so you must take greater care to sit straight. It is best to use a cushion to help you keep your weight down on the side of the straight leg. Spend more time breathing on your stiffer side to give it more stretch.

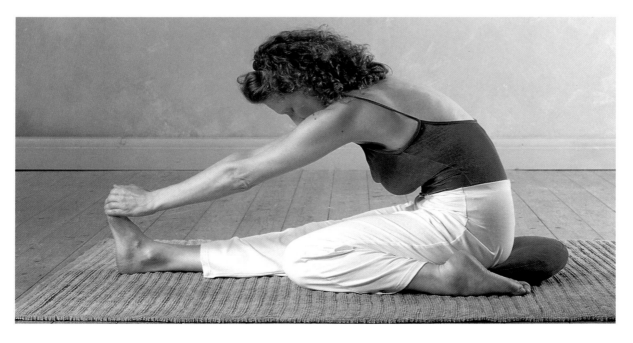

◁ Fold one leg and bring your foot beside your buttock, as in Virasana (48). Inhale and stretch your arms forward, keeping your shoulders level. Exhale and clasp your toes. Continue breathing in your lower back, extending more as you exhale. Release. Change legs and repeat.

71 "Easy" sage's pose (Marichyasana)

In this pose you are using one bent leg as a lever to further elongate the spine and release the hips. This is done first as a forward bend and then as a twist, in an easy version of the classic pose in which the bent arm entwines round the front of the knee.

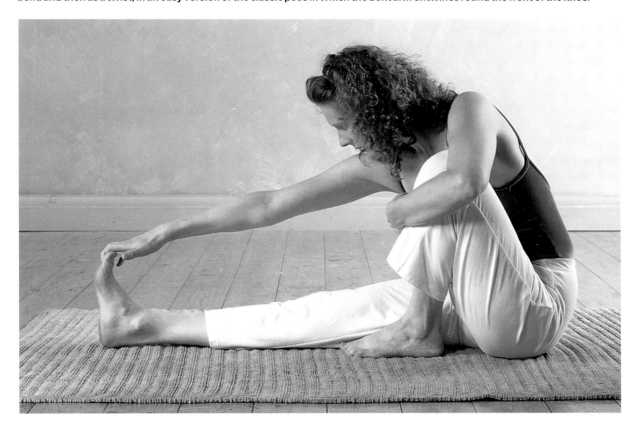

◁ **1** Bend one knee and bring your heel in against you, with your foot flat on the floor. Hold that knee close to your armpit. As you exhale, stretch forward to grasp the other foot with your free hand. If you are experienced in yoga, do the classic Marichyasana. Extend for a few breaths. Then change sides.

▷ **2** With your legs in the same position, finish this sequence with an open twist, placing your free hand on the floor behind you and stretching your spine up straight before you turn. Extend further with each out-breath, keeping your neck relaxed in the twist. Change sides.

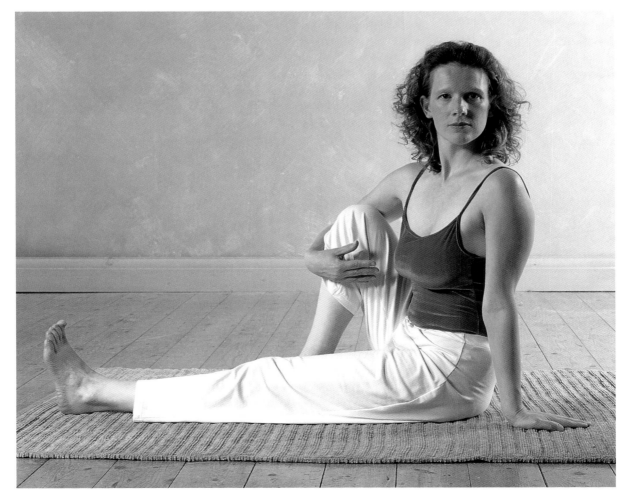

The plough and beyond

This sequence involves positions in which your trunk is inverted, or upside down. For this reason, you should avoid it when you have a period and as long as you feel that your internal energies are involved in clearing your womb and restoring its integrity.

In this sequence, movement and rhythm help you get into the Plough Pose (Halasana) and out of it into a forward bend more easily than by holding these two poses separately. Whether you are new to yoga or have some experience, the rolling plough sequence improves your skills at the stage where you are today. Rolling is also fun as well as stimulating for both you and your growing baby. If you can't get your buttocks off the floor at first, do not worry, just laugh and try the exercise again tomorrow.

72 The rolling plough sequence

The rolling plough sequence is an unconventional, but effective way of taking your feet over your head and extending backwards before stretching forward in a forward bend, which is already familiar to you. Your rolling sequence can be as small, or as acrobatic, as you wish or can have it. Never force it. Repeating a rhythmic backwards and forwards rolling movement will get you progressively into a full Plough without strain. This is a solid foundation for a shoulder stand, which you can then move to if you are experienced in yoga or may learn as part of a yoga class later.

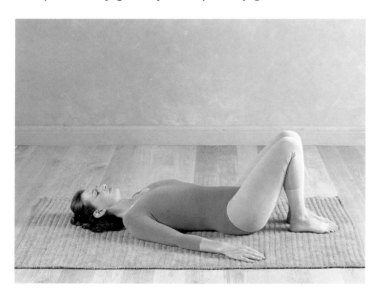

△ **1** Lie on the floor with your knees bent, feet flat and arms along your sides.

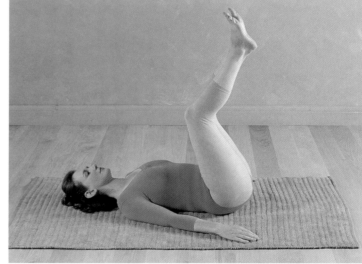

△ **2** Breathing in, lift your feet towards the ceiling, keeping your knees bent.

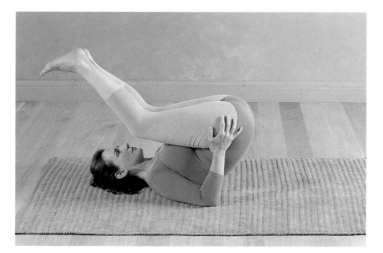

△ **3** Breathing out, bend your elbows and bring your hands to support your back, as you roll your hips backwards and up, bringing your knees towards your forehead. If doing this is difficult, move to 6, 7, 8.

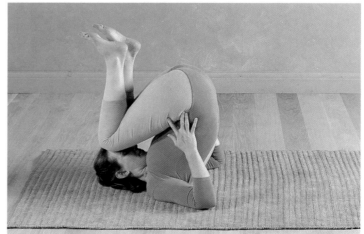

△ **4** If 3 is easy, continue rolling your knees to your forehead. If this is as much as you can do now, use your hands to support you as you lift your hips above your head, to get your spine vertical. Take a few breaths before moving to 6, 7, 8.

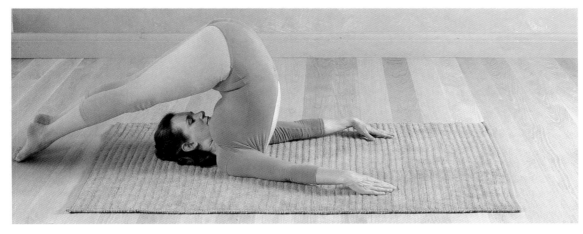

◁ **5** If 4 is easy, continue your rolling movement to straighten your legs, so that your feet rest on the floor behind you, keeping your arms down beside you. Stretch on an out-breath, inhale and start rolling your spine towards the floor, bending your knees.

▷ **6** Holding the back of your knees, keep the momentum of your roll to bring you to a sitting position. If you cannot roll easily, use your hands as a support to sit up.

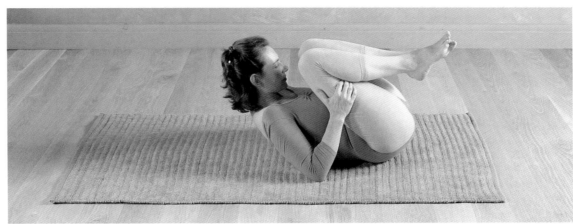

◁ **7** Sitting up is only a brief intermediate position in your rolling forward, extending your legs straight in front of you...

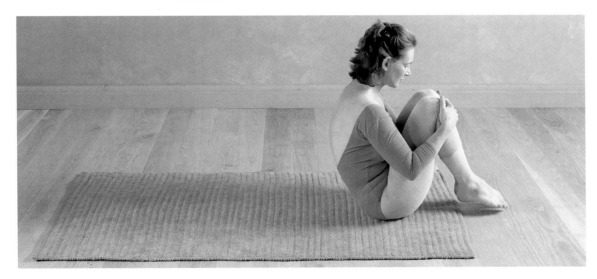

▷ **8** ...into a sitting forward bend. Stretch as you exhale and start rolling again backwards in the rolling sequence that suits you today. Get into a rhythm in which your breathing and movement allow you to roll and stretch in a relaxed way.

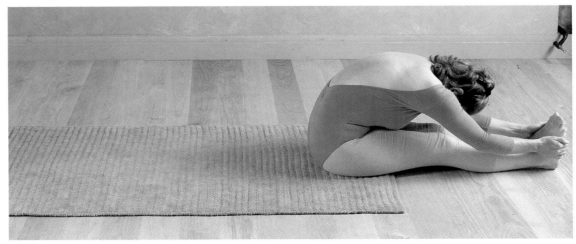

From relaxation to bliss

In the sequences that you have learnt and practised until now, stretching, breathing and relaxing have been equally important. You have probably become more aware of your breathing at all times, of your posture around your home and outside, with your baby and for yourself as a woman. Yoga has reminded you, in practice, how activity alternating with rest is the natural rhythm of life, as natural as breathing in and breathing out, or as day followed by night.

New mothers are often more tired from the constant attention they feel their babies need, day and night, than from lack of sleep. With relaxation, stress can be dissolved every day, as soon as it arrives. You can draw the strength you need to face unexpected challenges from reserves of deep rest. Progressively, as you become aware of your state of relaxation through regular practice of Shavasana (27), the Corpse Pose that renews you, the build-up of tension can be averted instantly, in any position you find yourself in. You learn to "let go", to release, to just be, in a not doing, not wanting state.

At this stage, you are ready to go from relaxation to meditation, which is one of the eight limbs of yoga. In the silence and stillness of relaxation, you can experience wholeness, peace and bliss. For new mothers, surrendering to unconditional love for their babies calls for an adequate source of self-nurture. Learning to "plug in" to the universal life-force at will in relaxation reminds us that this nurturing is infinite. "Plugging in" is simple and the more you practise it, the more rewarding it is for you, your baby and all your loved ones.

"It is vital to ask the spirits for their help or blessing, or you could wait for a long time! They never impose on us, but wait patiently to be consulted."

73 Deep rest

Every day, try to find a moment for relaxing into a deep rest. If your baby is asleep, extend your relaxation as long as you can after yoga. Being a rested mother comes top on your priority list. Bliss comes from this state of deep rest and an open heart.

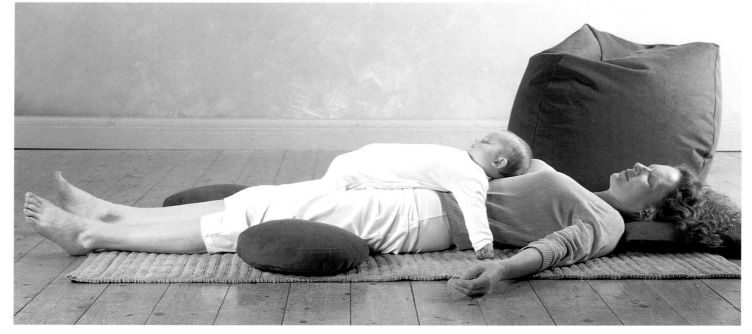

△ **Find a comfortable position and breathe deeply, concentrating on long breaths out. Let go and relax. Take time to return to activity.**

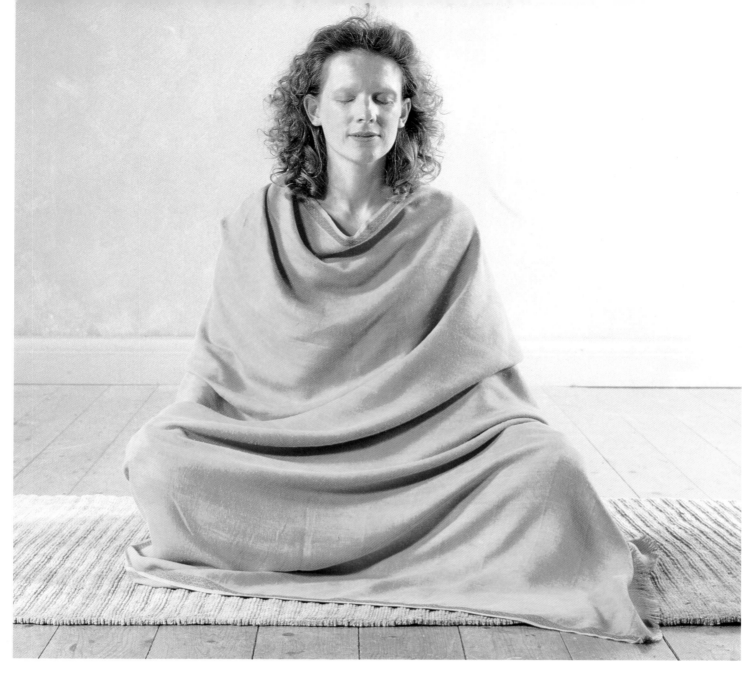

△ Sitting up with an erect spine is the ideal position to meditate, on the floor or on a chair. With practice, three long breaths will take you into this state – known in yoga as Ananda, which means "bliss". This is the meditative state, and the breath is the easiest tool with which to reach this state almost instantly. After a few more breaths, return to your external world, bringing your inner radiance with you. Refreshed and renewed, you can be "out there" again, ready for your baby.

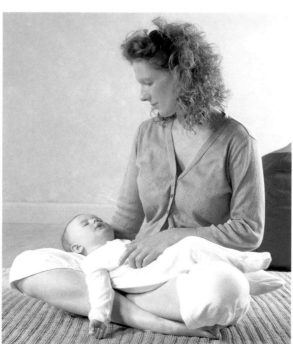

◁ If your baby is crying or unsettled, hold him or her gently and just be – in your heart centre, making contact again with the source of infinite nurturing inside you, letting yourself be held too.

Six months onwards

From now on you can add more classical asanas to your yoga sessions, whether or not you have joined a regular yoga class for further practice. If you have not practised before, it is worth finding the school of yoga that best suits your needs as a new mother.

different "schools" of yoga

There are several traditional schools of yoga, each focusing on different aspects of this vast subject. You may need to try out several different classes and teachers before you find the right ones for you. Yoga teachers are usually quite happy to let you join their classes for a week or two before signing on.

Ashtanga Vinyasa and Iyengar yoga are very physical and demanding. Viniyoga focuses on breath with gentle movement. Energy yoga focuses on moving energy through the body using classical breathing, cleansing techniques, visualization and meditation as well as asanas. The Sivananda,

Satyananda and Buddhist schools teach this more holistic type of yoga. Many yoga teachers are trained by national associations, which can put you in touch with teachers in your area.

Meanwhile, developing strength and stamina, while moving into more of the classical asanas, will give you an excellent foundation. The focus is still on poses that strengthen and "close" the pelvic and abdominal areas.

74 Tree pose (Vrkasana)

In this pose you should feel rooted, like a tree. Feel how the muscles on either side of your leg and trunk are working together, co-operating in the job of holding you upright and steady. Come out of the pose if you start to wobble. A "smaller" pose, well done, is better than wobbling in a more ambitious one! You can also stand against a wall to start with.

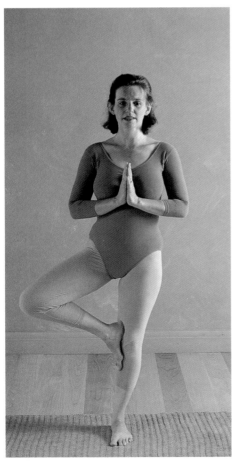

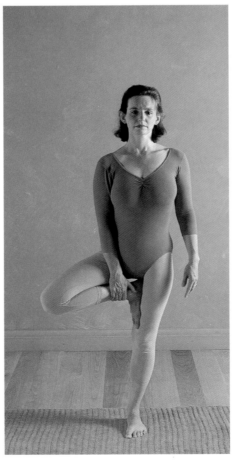

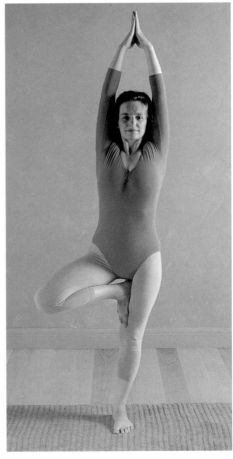

△ **1** Stand in Tadasana (28) and settle your body and breathing. Then bring one foot to rest on the inner side of your other leg, take your bent knee right out to the side, pull up your spine and join your palms in Namaste (10). Breathe freely. Change legs.

△ **2** Now for the classical pose: hold one foot and bring the sole against the opposite inner thigh, with the bent knee out to the side.

△ **3** Stand up tall and raise your straight arms slowly to the sides and then overhead, palms together, breathing in. Breathe deeply and hold the pose, coming out of it as gracefully as you went in. Repeat on the other side.

75 Standing seat (Utkatasana)

This asana is like sitting on an imaginary chair. Stand in Tadasana (28) and settle your body and breathing.

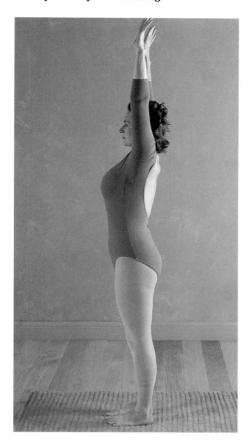

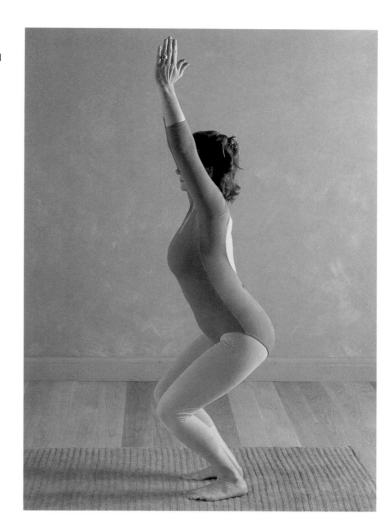

◁ **1** Breathing in, raise both your arms straight up overhead. Avoid arching the lower back. Stretch right through from your heels to your fingertips, and take a few deep breaths.

▷ **2** When you are ready, breathe out and bend your knees to "sit down", keeping your spine as nearly vertical as possible, until you are almost squatting, with your heels on the floor. Breathe deeply in the pose.

76 Standing forward bend (Padangusthasana)

This is an inverted pose, with your head lower than your heart. In contrast with the "Easy" Forward Bend (37) your feet are now together and your legs extended. Broaden the upper back and relax your head for a greater spinal stretch.

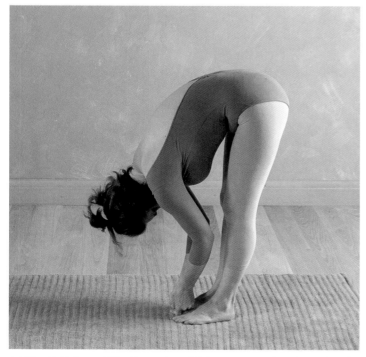

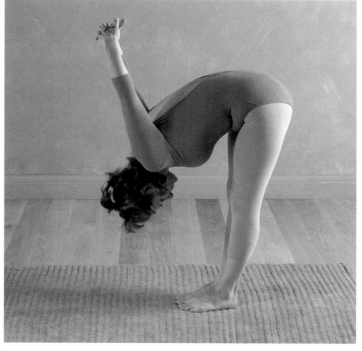

△**1** Stand in Tadasana (28) with your feet slightly apart. As you breathe out, bend forward and hold your big toes. Improve your position by looking up as you breathe in and relaxing down even more as you breathe out.

△**2** You can also practise the Chest Expansion exercise (as in 45 and 68, kneeling) in a standing forward bend.

Yoga for energy

As you are now following more and more the rise and fall of the flow of breath while you extend into the postures, you will be enjoying the special energy yoga brings. Rather than pushing your body to the limit in a workout, breathing in the postures as you can do them today – there is always more to come – stimulates all the systems of your physiology and increases your vital energy. Ups are not followed by downs after yoga. On the contrary, inner strength and enjoyment of life are constantly expanded.

77 Triangle pose (Trikonasana)

In this pose, the straight legs make a triangle. The back foot, firm on the floor, is your base as you stretch your spine vertebra by vertebra from the coccyx to the head, while you reach for the sky with a relaxed but straight arm.

▷ In the classical pose try to place your feet wider apart than for the "easy" version (36) – about the length of your leg – so there is more stretch. Practise first with your back to a wall, so that your head, shoulders and top hip brush against the wall as you stretch to the side and down. The point is to keep your spine elongating from the side, not to reach down. When you have a good "feel" for the position, practise away from the wall. Hold the position for several deep breaths, then repeat on the other side.

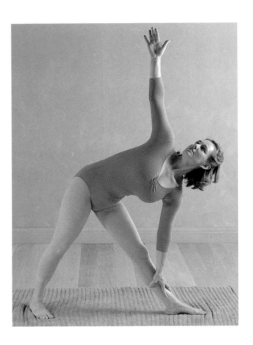

78 Downward-facing dog pose (Svanasana)

This is an inverted position, excellent for stretching and strengthening the whole body. The base of your spine is the apex of the pose, as you extend from the hands up your back and from your feet up your legs.

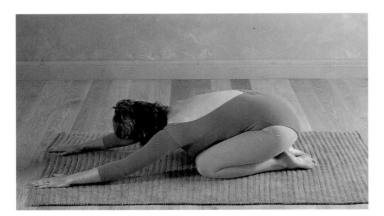

△ **1** Start in the Swan Pose (24), sitting on your heels and stretching your fingers forward. Prepare to turn your toes under.

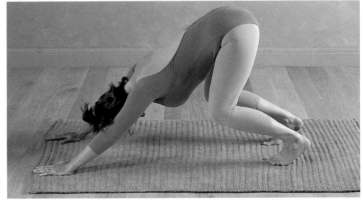

△ **2** Breathing in, raise your buttocks into the air, coming on to your toes, and extending the back. Push your buttocks back and up, bending your knees.

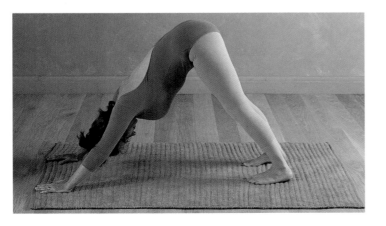

◁ **3** Progressively extend your heels towards the floor, straightening your legs. Make sure you release your neck and shoulders. With each exhalation, let your back grow longer and the top of your thighs stretch. When you are ready, breathe out and place your heels on the floor and your head between your arms, so that you are looking at your navel.

79 Upward-facing dog

This phase is an upward facing stretch with the spine bending backwards while the weight is on the wrists and feet. The two phases expand the Rhythmic Kneeling Sequence (47).

▷ From the Downward-facing Dog Pose, bring your hips down without moving your toes but lifting your heels, so that your body is suspended between your hands and your toes. Your head will come up. Gaze steadily forwards and breathe deeply. When you feel strong enough, and only then, lift your hips up into the Downward-facing Dog Pose. You can use the breath in these stretches: breathe out to face down and in to face up, in an easy swinging rhythm.

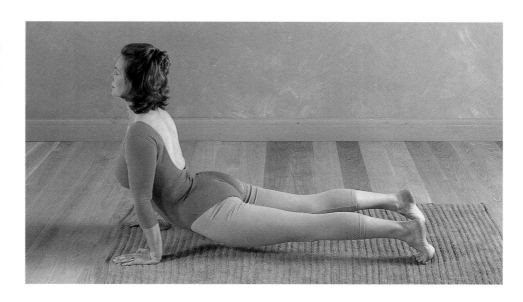

80 Equestrian pose

This pose continues the two phases of the Dog Pose as part of the classic Sun Salute. It is an intense toner of the legs and the hips as well as an energetic spinal stretch.

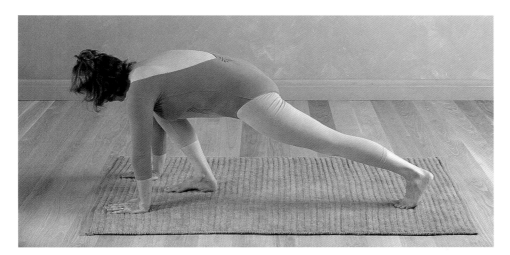

◁ **1** From the Downward-facing Dog Pose breathe in, as you swing your right foot forward between your hands. Lean hard to the side opposite your swinging leg, in order to get your chest out of the way.

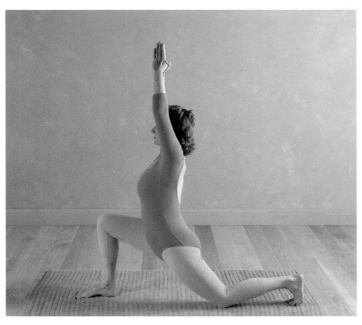

△ **2** With your left knee on the floor, inhale and raise your arms above your head while dropping your hips.

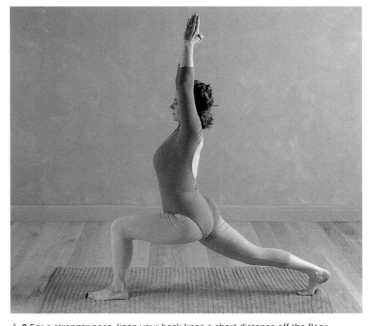

△ **3** For a stronger pose, keep your back knee a short distance off the floor. Breathe deeply, then return to the Downward-facing Dog Pose on an out-breath and swing the other foot forward, breathing in. Change sides, then relax.

Sunday afternoon yoga

What could be more nourishing to body and spirit than to practise yoga at home with your family – either indoors or outside in the garden on a warm day?

Make your yoga practice an exciting form of exercise, which you can share and enjoy with those around you. Everyone soon rises to the challenge, while yoga ceases to be something esoteric you do in your "yoga corner".

Walking Stretches

Cross-stride Walking (40) is an energetic and dynamic walking stretch which new mothers can practise in the park whilst remembering to breathe deeply.

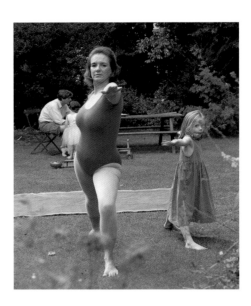

▷ To get into the swing, begin by walking normally, bringing your right arm and left leg forward together, then your left arm and right leg. Now change it, so that your left leg and arm come forward together, then your right leg and arm, in the Cross-stride Walk.

81 Warrior pose

Both the classic and the "Easy" Warrior Pose (57) can be done with a partner. Stand facing each other with the insteps of your right feet close together and your left legs stretched back. When Dad does yoga too, it can make a good show.

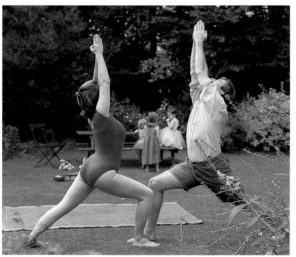

◁ **1** Keep your shins vertical as you sink your hips as low as possible, each adjusting the position of your back leg – the lower you sink down, the further away your back heel will be. Raise your arms triumphantly, with palms together. Breathe deeply and hold the pose.

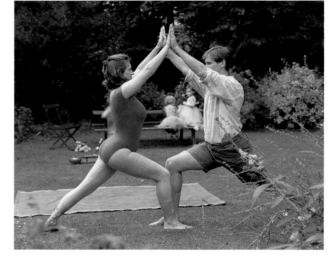

△ **2** You can "push hands" in the Warrior pose, to strengthen your arms and upper back.

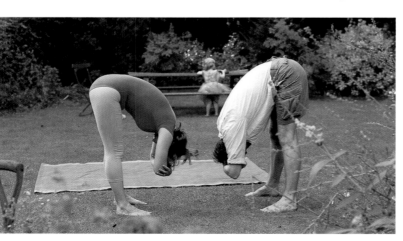

◁ **3** Step back and bow deeply to your partner in a Standing Forward Bend (76) with arms folded, before repeating the sequence with your left legs forward. Relax the neck and allow your spine to lengthen.

Floor exercises

The whole family can enjoy sitting poses on the grass in the summer. The Rolling Plough Sequence (72) is always good fun, even if it ends in a heap of bodies.

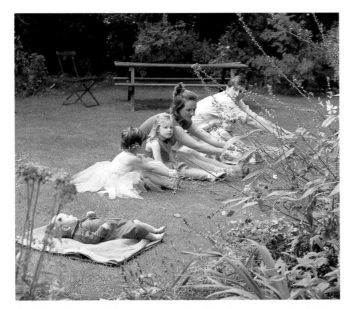

△ **1** Line up for a Seated Forward Bend (Paschimottanasana) (69) stretching forward with straight legs.

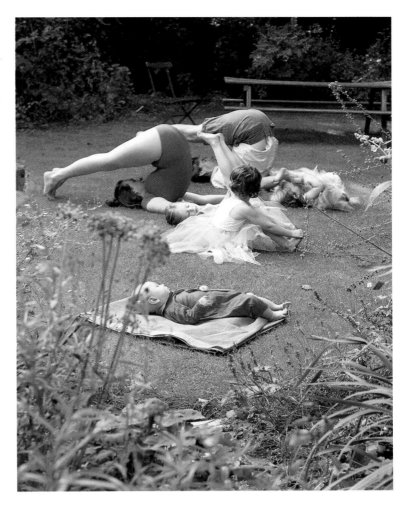

▷ **2** Roll back and up into the plough pose.

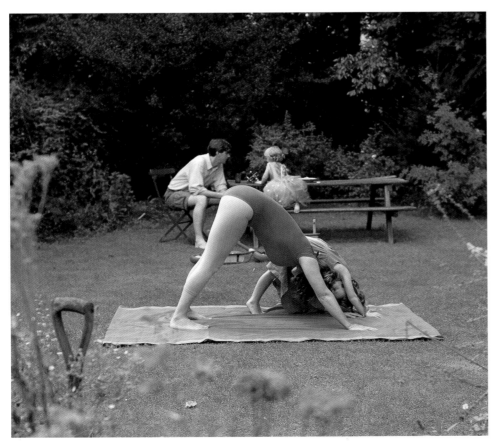

△ **3** Doing your yoga practice outdoors can be invigorating. The Downward-facing Dog Pose (78) is always popular with older children while your baby is asleep.

Togetherness time

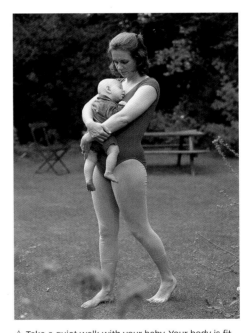

△ Take a quiet walk with your baby. Your body is fit and strong, your mind clear and rested, and your heart full of love. This "walking meditation" can be a celebration of your baby, or you can turn to it for help in calming both you and your baby on difficult days. That's the beauty of yoga. It promotes well-being at every level in your life, just as it is, from day to day.

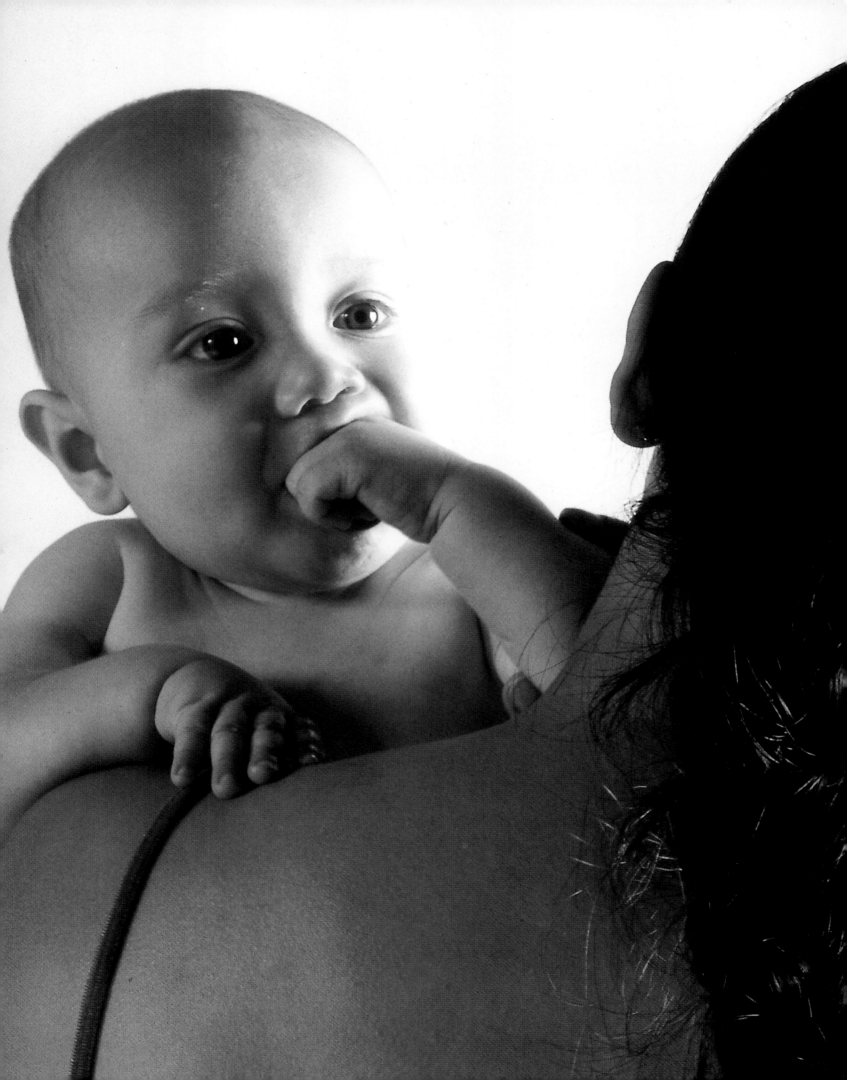

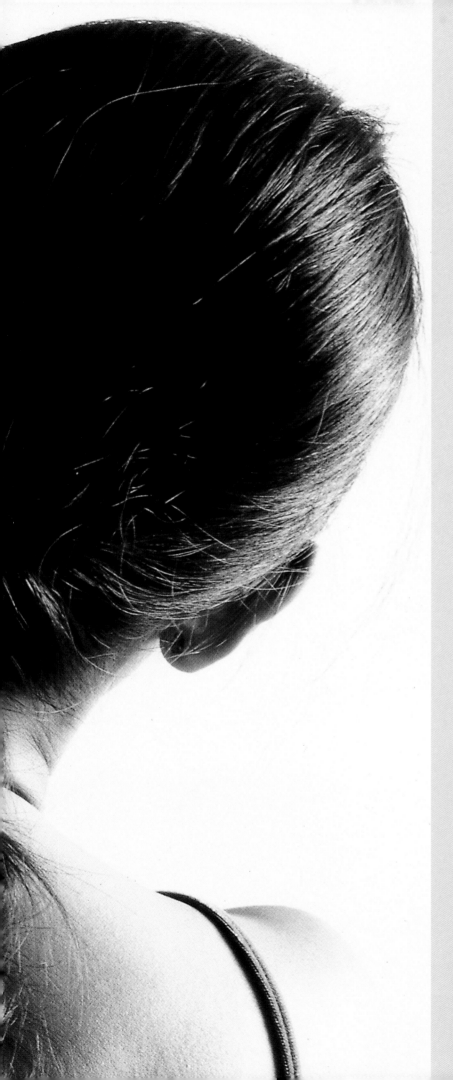

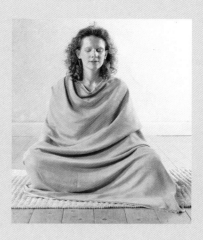

good
practice

Many of the physical dysfunctions that afflict

new mothers can be eased or put right with

deep breathing in specific yoga postures.

A strong, elastic pelvic floor, good posture

and better circulation are fundamental for

women's well-being. While yoga stimulates

the body's internal systems, relaxation can

unfold its self-healing capacity.

First period routine

Up to now you have been working within a particular cycle – that of pregnancy, birth and recovery. Prenatal yoga emphasizes "opening" poses to facilitate the growth and birth of the baby. Postnatal yoga then emphasizes "closing" and strengthening poses to regain pre-pregnancy pelvic health.

The day your first period arrives is the start of a new cycle – that of the monthly "opening" to release waste products from the womb. Here is a suggested routine – a "rite of passage" – to mark this change. It can also be used each month in the first two days of your period. In the yoga tradition, inverted poses are not to be practised during the full flow of menstruation.

Shavasana (with knees bent) (27)

This is the end of a cycle that started when your baby was conceived. Now your baby is here. You are bleeding again. Relax to enter this transition.

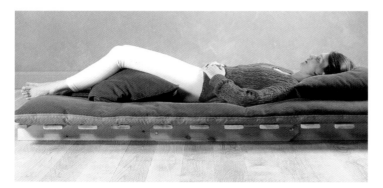

△ Start by lying down on your back on a rug or bed, with your knees bent and your arms loose on each side of your body. Inhale and exhale deeply several times, making a greater contact between your waist and the floor or bed each time you exhale. Make sure your buttock muscles are relaxed after you tighten and release your pelvic floor muscles, inhaling and exhaling in a rhythm that suits you. Then relax.

Side stretch (9)

Go back to this early gentle stretch to elongate the lower spine and soothe your pelvic nerves.

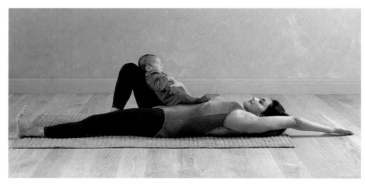

△ Stretch from your heel to your fingertips for a few seconds as you inhale and start exhaling, then release at the end of the exhalation. Repeat a few times, then change sides.

Forward bend (2) (62)

This combined stretch and bend can also be practised kneeling on a cushion if you find standing too demanding. It brings oxygenated blood to the pelvis as you breathe deeply and freely, releasing all tension on the out-breath.

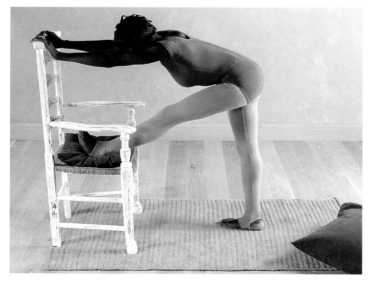

△ **1** Stretch up and forward from your hips, opening the lower back. Breathe deeply, pulling your stomach muscles in towards the spine and drawing up your pelvic floor.

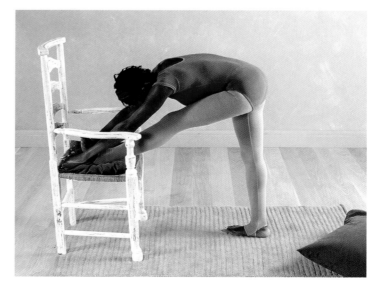

△ **2** Release all muscles on your out breath. This is the opposite of Reverse Breathing (1). Repeat a few times.

Rhythmic kneeling sequence (47)

After stretching in the Rhythmic Kneeling Sequence (47) enjoy resting in the Child Pose (67), earthing and drawing up your inner strength.

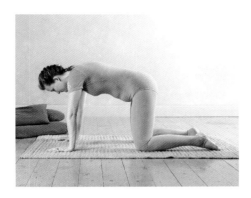

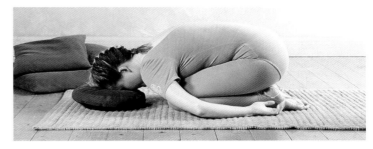

◁ **1** Practise the Rhythmic Kneeling Sequence slowly as this will help to loosen your whole back.

△ **2** Relax in a kneeling forward bend, the Child Pose, with a cushion under your forehead, breathing freely.

82 Half bound angle pose (Janu Sirsasana)

This classic yoga pose is most helpful to hold the womb in its optimal position. During your period, breathe freely to relax the perineum in the pose.

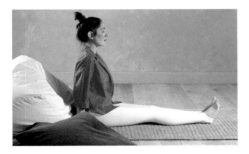

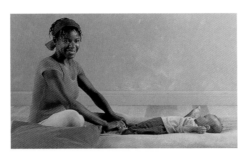

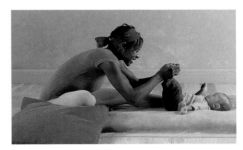

△ **1** Start by sitting in Dandasana (51), with your back and legs straight. Propping yourself up with your hands on the sides of your body if needed, relax your lower back and abdominal muscles on each exhalation for a few breaths. Feel a downward flow of energy towards the floor.

△ **2** Then, keeping one leg straight, bend your other knee and bring the foot against the inside of the straight leg as close to the perineum as possible. Put a cushion under your bent knee if needed. Breathe deeply, drawing in your pelvic floor muscles as you inhale, relaxing totally as you exhale.

△ **3** Bending from the hips and elongating your spine as much as you can, extend forward, keeping your shoulders and head relaxed. Keep your weight down on the hip of the bent leg on each exhalation. Hold for a few breaths, sit back in Dandasana, then change sides.

Legs up the wall (5)

Make the most of your yoga breathing to start your cycle anew and reduce or eliminate pre-menstrual tension and period pains.

Sitting breathing, relaxation and meditation

As you sit quietly, undoing any tension in your body and mind, explore the infinite potential of the breath to enhance your reproductive health.

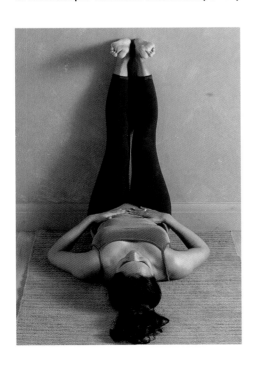

◁ With your hands on your lower abdomen, breathe as deeply as you can, drawing in your pelvic floor muscles as you inhale, relaxing completely as you exhale. Keep your legs relaxed against the wall and feel how their weight helps you breathe deeper into your lower back. If you wish, explore the feeling of "opening" with this breathing.

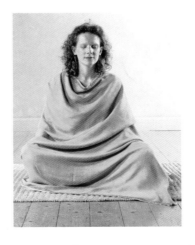

Sit comfortably, against a wall with cushions if this is better for you, or on a chair, so as to keep your back upright. Practise the Alternate Nostril Breathing (2) for a couple of minutes, to clear your mind and centre you. Drop your lower jaw and relax along the vertical axis from the crown of your head to your perineum. You will begin to feel aligned, toned and yet open and relaxed at the same time. Feel the palms of your hands soft whilst your arms are resting on your lap. Feel where you are, right now, in your self as you return to menstruation. Acknowledge any emotions that you have about it and how mixed they can be. Feel them, and let go of them. Find your core self within and acknowledge your feminine energy and its transformation through pregnancy and birth. Feel grateful and blessed for your baby, and the person that you are now becoming.

Expanding your yoga practice

The "core" of yoga is outlined at the start of this book: that is breath, relaxation, awareness, stretching – especially through the spine – and strengthening. This core remains, however simple or complicated your yoga practice may be. Three sample routines follow, showing how your practice may develop as you grow stronger, while still maintaining the yoga core. You can invent hundreds of permutations of your own, following the same general plan.

You will see that the simpler exercises continue alongside the more advanced ones. When you plan to practise a particular classical posture, you will choose simpler movements of a similar type – backward or forward bending, twists or balances – to use as a preliminary warm-up for the more testing stretches.

Let yoga breathing, relaxation, awareness and posture become part of your life. Your whole attitude will change because you are coming from a space that is more centred, less fragmented; more welcoming, less anxious.

A sample practice for birth to six weeks

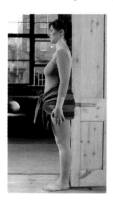

1

◁ **Tadasana (28)**
Start with aligning your spine so that you become aware of your posture after pregnancy.

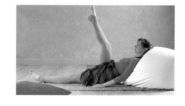

2

△ **With reverse breathing (1)**
Use this breathing exercise while in Tadasana to tone and strengthen your entire trunk.

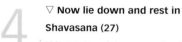

3

◁ **Then circle your feet**
The ligaments and muscles of your feet and ankles need strengthening after your change in weight.

4

▽ **Now lie down and rest in Shavasana (27)**
This may complete your session, if it is a very short one. You can continue next time you have a few suitable moments, starting with a short rest, or carry on now.

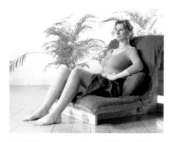

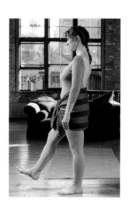

5

△ **Abdominal and pelvic floor muscles, lying down (12)**
Have cushions or a beanbag near you.

6

▽ **Basic kneeling sequence (24, 25, 26)**
Spend some time on this sequence, then rest. Stop here, or carry on a little longer…

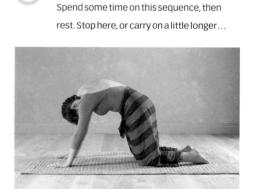

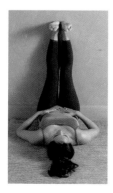

7

◁ **Legs up the wall (5)**
Rest when you have breathed deeply with each knee bent in turn.

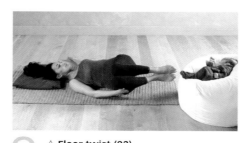

8

△ **Floor twist (23)**
A good way to ease and stretch your lower spine, even if you had a Caesarian section.

9

▽ **Final Rest: Shavasana (27)**
This relaxation should last longer than the rests between exercises, so keep warm.

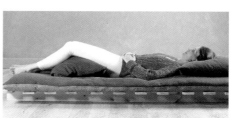

A sample practice for six to twelve weeks

You can use some of the exercises suggested for birth to six weeks to prepare for stronger stretches. Reverse breathing (1) is essential to tone your abdominal muscles in depth. Whatever your stretch level is, make sure you pay full attention to using the breath in your yoga practice.

1 ▽ **Alternate nostril breathing (2)**
Sit on a firm chair, ready for the next sequence.

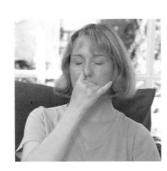

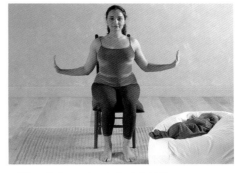

2 △ **Sun wheel stretch (16)**

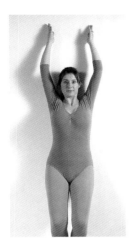

3 ◁ **Standing against a wall (32)**
Standing tall with your whole spine against the wall, practise Reverse Breathing (1) with your arms lifted.

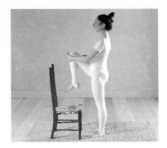

4 △ **"Easy" tree pose (Vrkasana) (38)**
After practising this pose, your baby may like some attention, so choose something you can have fun with together. Remember to pause and breathe deeply before picking up your baby.

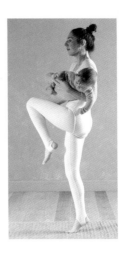

5 ◁ **Cross-stride prancing (41)**
This continues the high-stepping of your previous pose, but is active and energetic. It also has a twisting movement.

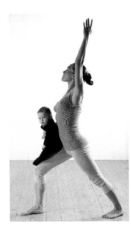

6 ◁ **Walking warrior pose (42)**
After this you will both need a rest!

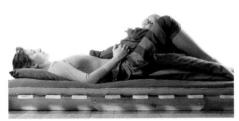

7 △ **Shavasana (27)**
When you decide to continue with your session you will recall that you have done no floor poses so far.

8 ▽ **Basic kneeling sequence (24, 25, 26)**
This is always good to do, as it makes the spine flexible and releases tension.

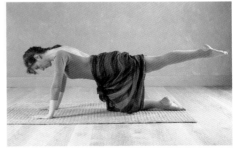

9 ▽ **Rhythmic kneeling sequence (47)**

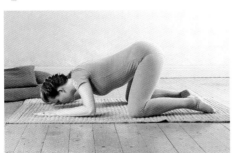

10 △ **Child pose (see 67)**
Breathe deeply into the back of your lungs and your lower abdomen.

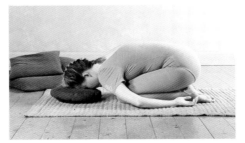

11 ▽ **Final relaxation: Shavasana (27)**

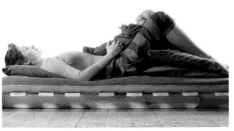

A sample practice for three to six months

1 ▽ **Reverse breathing, second stage, in Shavasana (3 and 27)**

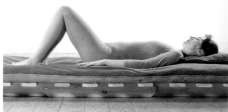

2 △ **Reverse breathing (1) while raising the hips (33)**
This is a backbend.

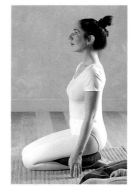

3 ◁ **Vajrasana (43)**

4 ▽ **Chest expansion (45)**
This is a forward bend, after the backbend.

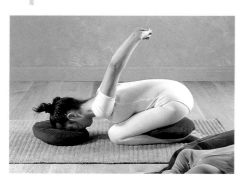

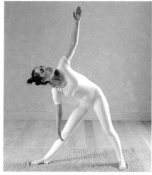

5 △ **Kneeling twist with elbow rotations (46)**
The basics have been attended to, so now for something new.

6 ▽ **"Easy" sage's pose (Marichyasana) (71)**

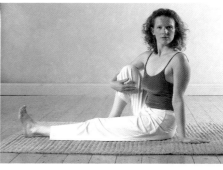

7 ▽ **Rest in child pose (see 67)**

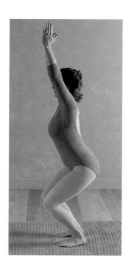

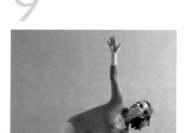

8 △ **"Easy" triangle pose (36)**
Repeat a few times on each side, to prepare for the classical version.

9 ▽ **Triangle pose (Trikonasana) (77)**

10 ◁ **Standing seat (Utkatasana) (75)**
Elongate the lower part of your spine as you breathe deeply in this pose.

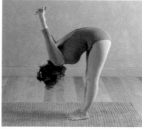

11 △ **Standing forward bend (Padangusthasana) (76)**
Perhaps you have time for a few more poses while your baby is peaceful. If so, you could add the Downward- and Upward-facing Dog (78 and 79) and "Easy" Warrior Pose (57). If not, don't worry!

12 ▽ **Alternate nostril breathing (2)**
Sit cross-legged for this.

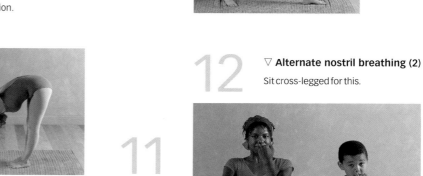

Useful addresses and thanks

For advice on postnatal matters:
Birthlight
7 Essex Close
Cambridge CB4 2DW, UK
Tel (01223) 362288

Yoga for mothers, with specialized teachers:
Birthlight / Yoga Biomedical Trust UK
60 Great Ormond Street
London WC1N 3HR, UK
Tel (0207) 419 7195

General yoga classes, with trained teachers:
British Wheel of Yoga
Central Office, 1 Hamilton Place
Boston Road, Sleaford
Lincolnshire NG34 7ES, UK
Tel (01529) 306 851

For information and referral to support groups:
National Childbirth Trust (NCT)
Alexandra House, Oldham Terrace
London W3 6NH, UK
Tel (0208) 922 8637

**Childbirth Education Association
of Australia (Brisbane) Inc**
P.O. Box 208
Chermside 4032
Australia
Tel (07) 3359 9725

Postpartum Support International
(for worldwide referral)
9271 Kellog Avenue
Santa Barbara, CA 93117
United States
Tel (USA) 805 967 7636

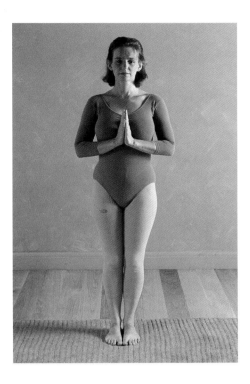

Author's Acknowledgements

Many thanks to Alison and Charlie who kindly opened their home and garden to be photographed. Thanks to Doriel Hall for spurring me to turn my classes into books and co-writing this one as a "new" grandmother. Her great expertise and precision have been invaluable in directing the photography and writing the first draft. Thanks also to Christine Hanscomb for the outstanding photographs and to Sue Duckworth for not only being an expert stylist but a caring one too. Thanks to Debra Mayhew for her excellent editorial assistance as well as her skills in creating a happy productive team to implement the vision for this book. Thanks to Andrea Wilson in London and Sally Lomas in Cambridge for pioneering Birthlight classes; to my co-directors of Birthlight for unfailing support; to Robin Monro for giving a venue and recognition to postnatal yoga at the London Yoga Therapy Centre.

My gratitude also goes to many teachers and also to all the Birthlight mothers who have helped me to refine the approach presented in this book since my children were born. My warmest thanks are to my whole family for their love and inspiration. Thanks to Drake for his heartfelt wonder of birth shared with our Amazonian and Hawaiian "families". It is my sincere hope that this book may help towards alleviating postpartum depression and to create what Robin Lim called "wellness after the baby's birth".

Thank you to the models

Many thanks to the mothers and their families who gave up their time to take part in this book. All have benefited from the yoga exercises featured here. Katrien Asakura-Vanassche and Kojo Asakura with Koo (4 years old) and Kenji (10 weeks); Karyn Barnes and Felicity Yeo with Lauryn (4 weeks); Ros Belford with Ismene (6 months); Hayley Brewis with Annabel (3 weeks); Nina Cooke with Louis (2 months); Sally Davis and Andrew Hill with Kate (4 years), Zoey (2 years) and Zan (4 months); Claudia Dossena with Isaac (20 weeks); Charlotte Forbes with Elsa (14 weeks); Pam Ha-Stevenson with Joshua (6 months); Victoria Lampert with Harry (6 months); Sam Marshall with Molly (4 months); Carol Morgan with Benjamin and Joseph (twins, 3 months); Tracy Rodericks with Aidan (7 weeks); Mai and Rob Ward with Ruby and Honor (twins, 5 months); Sarah Wood with Harrison (4 ½ months); Safuriat Yesufu and Rob with Morton (3 months) and Emile (4).

Index

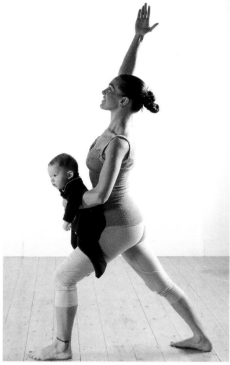

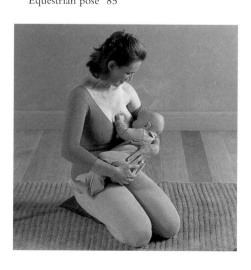

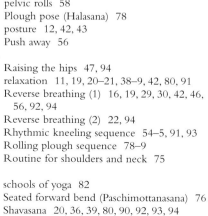

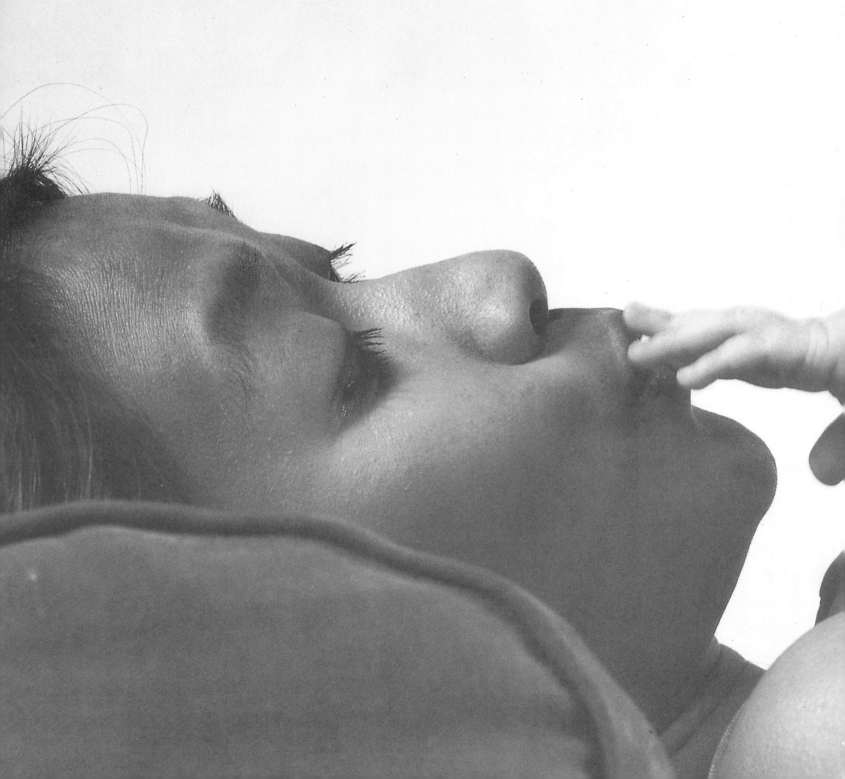